Abraham Z. Shoshani

EXPERIENCING YOUR POTENTIAL

For my parents, **Hannah and Zrubavel Shoshani,** of blessed memory
For my brother, **Shlomo Shoshani,** of blessed memory

ABRAHAM Z. SHOSHANI
EXPERIENCING YOUR POTENTIAL
Following Feldenkrais' Work
The Elusive Border between Learning, Psychology, and Art

TRANSLATED BY FELICE KAHN ZISKEN

DEKEL PUBLISHING HOUSE

EXPERIENCING YOUR POTENTIAL
Following Feldenkrais' Work
The Elusive Border between Learning, Psychology, and Art

ISBN: 965-7178-06-1
EAN: 978-965-7178-06-5
Printed in Israel

For information contact:
Dekel Publishing House
P.O.Box 45094
Tel Aviv 61450, Israel
dekelpbl@netvision.net.il
Tel: +972-3-6045379
Fax:+972-3-5440824

In collaboration with the Center for Culture of the East
Jerusalem, Israel

Translated by Felice Kahn Zisken
Designed by Studio KavGraph

Copyright © 2006 by Dr. Abraham Z. Shoshani

All rights reserved. No part of this book may by reproduced or transmitted in any form or any means, electronic or mechanical, including photocopying, recording or by any information storage and retrieval system, without permission in writing from Dekel Publishing House

TABLE OF CONTENTS

Foreword: Prof. Zvi Lam – Hebrew University, Jerusalem 6

Preface: 7

Introduction 9

Chapter One: The Interactive Action of the Nervous System 13

Chapter Two: Potency and Movement 19

Chapter Three: Psychic Integration and the Concept of Mind 23

Chapter Four: Learning and Experiencing 33

Chapter Five: A State of Disorder 51

Chapter Six: Vocal Expression and its Centrality in Knowing

and Experiencing 77

Chapter Seven: Art as Cure 97

Appendix: Biography of Dr. Moshe Feldenkrais 110

FOREWORD

In *Experiencing Your Potential*, Dr. Shoshani confronts a challenging topic. For this he enlists, his rich experience in mentoring students in various art disciplines and his accumulated knowledge of neurophysiology, psychology, philosophy, and education.

Dr. Shoshani's preparation of the student is not a training technique. His every word is charged with profound educational meaning. The student learns more than the different implementations, he learns about himself as performer, according to the path that the author has outlined for him.

The essence of Dr. Shoshani's work can be summarized in his differentiation of four basic components in scientific activity and artistic self-expression:

1. Experiencing of the self as fully involved in doing and acting.
2. The feeling of control over one's actions
3. The individual's involvement in a goal which is clarified as it is realized
4. The feeling of being directed by necessity and the desire to continue despite the difficulties.

This work offers thinking challenges to the interested reader and inspiration and guidance to anyone involved in performance education.

Prof. Zvi Lam
Hebrew University, Jerusalem

PREFACE

My career as an artist and educator was influenced by the lessons of Dr. Moshe Feldenkrais. The heart of the matter appears to lie in clarifying the intention and realizing it in movement, such that there is no separation between the intention and the movement, and that in the eyes of the performer the two are perceived as one. Dr. Feldenkrais taught us that the unity and simplicity of the movement are the basis of its beauty, both in the feeling of the performer and in the eyes of the beholder.

Moshe Feldenkrais devised numerous lessons composed of series of movements that train us to recreate within ourselves learning processes free of any outside influence or unclear reason. These processes, accumulated over many years, could contribute towards changes in how we adapt to the field of gravity, as well as in how we perceive ourselves and our fellow man.

In this book I discuss, among other subjects, the connections between Dr. Feldenkrais' work and works of other experts in the fields of neurophysiology, psychology, education, philosophy, and more, coupled with my own extensive experience in teaching various artistic disciplines.

My work has shown that the concept of mind and its unity are also connected with the various neuromotor systems, and therefore a connection can be made between the imaginary artistic world and the learning processes, which are none other than the building of the mind and bringing it from the potential to the actual.

The psychophysical unity of man is reflected in artistic activity, in which the physical reality and the symbolic reality frequently combine, and this is the moment of grace when the idea of unity of the mind, which in the past drew the attention of numerous researchers, is brought to fruition.

I had the privilege to be among Dr. Feldenkrais' students in the 1960s and 1970s in Israel, and to this day I practice his methods as part of my daily regime.

Dr. Abraham Z. Shoshani
Jeruslem, March 2006

INTRODUCTION

Can one build a model with a conceptual system that helps us understand both learning processes and the processes of artistic expression on the stage? Is there a connection between these two processes? In the natural sciences, for example, the concept of energy applies to all physical existence, which explains its depth. There is also a homogeneous *weltanschaung*, a perspective that all visual phenomena are of the same type. Can one, with the processes of learning and artistic expression, do what "science" does, namely, deconstruct the whole into its important elements so that their inter-relationships and their relationship to the whole are revealed? The whole, in our case, is the human being who is connected in different ways to his environment, to one extent or another, and sometimes in extreme cases, cut off from this connection.

It seems to me that, at their best, the art of performance and the learning process clarify the individual's connection with himself and with his environment. In my opinion, work with the student who aspires to be an artist or researcher should aim to expand and deepen the range of listening to what is happening within, by reducing **"parasitic forces"** which are often connected to the search for love and value and with taking on tasks too early, that is to say, without sufficient clarification of internal experiences that are intertwined with the studied and performed material.

These "parasitic forces" are physically expressed in the individual's self-imposed limitations, in excluding positions and movements that he profoundly feels may prevent love and appreciation. Reducing these forces may result in both a richer use of self and a clarification of emotional and cognitive processes that was impossible earlier.

In my experience, after reducing the "parasitic forces", the student feels a sense of wholeness with himself and is more alert to what happens in himself and in his environment. He is in a state of inner growth and flourishing, which brings great satisfaction. In my opinion, both the performer and the student should be involved in processes **that become clearer as they are performed** and not be involved in "efforts" to "perform" activities which actually stop the process and prevent spontaneous action (see below the definition of "effort" and "spontaneity").

One can generalize and say that the spontaneous act is an act in which the ego is not involved in "how" but rather, is involved interactively in the feeling of solidarity with self or with the character personified on the stage (in the case of the actor).

The character is not constructed in a contrived intellectual way in response to what has to be done, but with imagination and internalization which bring about a motor sensation and response. (See below for a discussion of "solidarity" and "interactivity").

In this frame of mind, the artist has a sense of capability and free will, despite the objective constraints of text, staging, and requisite props. Technically, the problems of performance on the stage may arise when one tries to compensate by using different parts of the periphery of the body. This "compensation" conceals the problems of the body's "posture" which influence the quality of breathing and doing.

Clearly, "posture" is not a static but a dynamic concept that reflects mood and tendency and the question of how posture is acquired is of great significance. (See below for definition of the terms "posture" and the "sense of free will".)

I believe that if we pay attention to the emotional-motor reality, we lessen the need for "compensation" and at the same time elicit the student's clarification process.

The student may reach a level of differentiation - for example, when he solves a question, says these lines, or plays that piece, he knows if he is negating himself and assuming tasks that ultimately he knows he cannot perform. Or perhaps the process which occurs within is simply and directly expressed in the process of performing and learning.

In addition, when we consider the emotional-motor reality in stage performance, we clarify and enrich self-image and the performer will then also have a clearer feeling of the addressee and be able to naturally project his voice to the audience.

It seems to me that in successful learning, the student learns to look inward and express himself simply and directly, which also enhances his connection with the environment and the understanding that he has control over the time dimension and is not forced into a foreign and mechanical external rhythm.

In my work I have found that when a student enriches his own body image, his sense of space also improves and consequently, he becomes master of time, **time that he actually creates.** In this state of clarification, flexibility and inner harmony, there is opportunity for authentic imaginative expression that sometimes touches this abstract quality which is the core of artistic performance and innovative thinking.

In conclusion, we should be involved with processes and not with results, not determining what is to be implemented, but rather, guiding the student so that he knows something he did not know before – in a way that suits him.

By eliminating rigid, a priori positions, we create a more flexible and richer use of self and thus, a sensitive, flexible and rich reality is developed in the course of performance and learning which transforms the process into something alive and dynamic; the materials are adapted while the unity of consciousness and experience is preserved.

Below I will discuss the elements of the neuro-motor system that enable the organism to function in harmony as one whole with the environment.

In the learning process of basic skills such as sitting, walking and standing, the parent's attempt to demand a premature response or overprotect the child can undermine these elements and delegitimize the learning process - the child's confident movement to the **unknown** with his inner wholeness intact.

In the coming chapters, I will present the evolutionary processes through which man has reached a more potent state as well as the concept of "mind" which, I believe, is connected with the concept of meaning and intention and the ability to find an appropriate response to outer stimuli. The ability to learn which, in my opinion, is inherent in man, can be jumbled into a state of disorder whose repair must involve regaining the ability of solidarity-interactivity action.

CHAPTER ONE
The Interactive Action of the Nervous System

The contribution of the nervous system to the animate world is manifest at its highest level in the live organism's response to the external world. Two related principles characterize this response:
1. Interactivity
2. Solidarity within self

The animal that receives all the stimuli from its environment simultaneously functions with orderly actions in the time dimension. If all the animal's actions were simultaneous, the resulting chaos would make the animal's continued existence impossible. The animal's functioning means the inhibition of certain responses for the sake of other responses. "Inhibition" is defined as coordination of the different neuro-motor components so that the animal's actions are appropriately orderly according to its need for survival. Once more, interactivity means coordination of the different components to ensure the animal's continued existence as an intact whole organism.

These processes of inhibition are usually inherent in the animal and no one can know who inhibits or elicits this or that neuron at a given moment; rather, a quasi-predetermined plan serves the animal's continued survival in its environment.

As to solidarity, we can see that if the animal's leg is injured in a specific place, the response will be twofold. One response, the animal will lift the injured leg from the ground and two, the animal will flee from the place of injury as **one intact** entity. This illustrates the phenomena of solidarity or of the animal's identifying as a whole organism with the wounded leg.

The effector neuron (the nerve cell) that activates the muscles can receive pulses from different and even antagonistic sources and yet, the animal functions in nature in an orderly way in the dimension of time. A series of reflexes activate the animal as one entity. The body's anti-gravitational tone also connects to reflexes that enable the animal to stand and respond to the environment while its eyes always return to the state in which the retina remains in a permanent position, both vertically and horizontally.

The nervous system is at its peak in the integration of series of segments that work together with each other. We can see here the principle of unity within multiplicity. Or, formulated differently, the main task of the central nervous system is to send pulses to the muscles that will cause the body to move effectively as a whole.

The reflexes are not refined and precise and have quasi-pre-prepared responses to situations that are more-or-less known beforehand. In more developed animals, a conditioned reflex with a more precise response can be created; for example, the distinction between a circle and an ellipse or the ability to recognize different sounds.

In the autonomous nervous system that is composed of the sympathetic and parasympathetic systems, there is also an antagonistic adjustment between the parts, that is to say, the activity of one makes the activity of the second impossible. This antagonistic adjustment exists in the animal in nature and serves its continued existence. We will see later that this is not always the case with human beings. Man is meant to activate the two antagonistic parts in the same period in time, something that physically reflects contradictory processes that exist psychically in the human being.

Clearly a simultaneous functioning of antagonistic parts does not serve any purpose.

The sympathetic part functions in response to threat and enables the animal to fight or flee (or freeze in place) and the parasympathetic part facilitates rest and recovery and the organism's return to balance (homeostasis).

When the animal freezes in place, the inhibition of the extensor muscles facilitates their functioning with redoubled energy so that it can flee. I will discuss this trait of induction later.

The stages of the reflex response are as follows:
a. A response to avoid injury from stimulation, for example, closing one's eyes to the stimulus of an intense light.
b. The organism adapts to a return to the state of balance – when the eyes are closed, the dilated pupils expand – which makes seeing in normal conditions possible.

If we consider the example of an external threat, then the first stage of response is contracting the flexors, a fast pulse, holding one's breath. In the second stage, contracting the flexors muscles sends a signal of confidence to the nervous system – something that causes a lowered pulse and more regular breathing. This signal of confidence stems from the fact that in a fall, the contraction of the flexors protects the head and the internal organs; this developed in evolution.

Chapter One

Until now, we have listed two elements that characterize the animal's response to the external world, but in more developed animals with teleceptors, there is an additional element - one sensor's influence on the other, strengthening the process for the final cause. The cause can be prey, coupling etc. Here the basis of time begins to be formed, since the animal moves to a future cause and adapts to the changing consequences in efforts to reach its goal.

When a specific experience is acquired, the entire situation is enforced, even if there is only a partial presentation. This characteristic, vital for survival, facilitates a simultaneous response to menace or the mating that guarantees the race's continued existence.

The teleceptors control how the muscles are used; they are also widely represented in the cortex and therefore enable the organism to present itself as a whole. The teleceptors, connected to both the cortex and the body, create an entity with a more complete and refined solidarity.

This is the beginning of the creation of mind, since there is a differentiation between two different informations, one kinesthetic and the other stemming from the teleceptors, that reflect the same reality. It is interesting to note, in this context, that in the course of evolution, the muscle "birthed" the nerve and the nerve "birthed" the brain. The muscle seems to have had enough "mind" to know that a nerve and then later a brain would be necessary for coping with reality. Development was characterized in that, among other things, more "commanders" gave instructions, more or less to the same "performers".

It is important to remember that the muscle is both receptor and effector. It enters information into the system and also implements the high hierarchic orders.

With the development of life in evolution and the building of the central nervous system and the teleceptors, the possibility of choosing means towards the realization of goals was also created, or in other words, the possibility of seeing cause and effect. Interestingly, this seems connected to the one-directionality of the central nervous system (time is also one-directional).

In contrast, there are cells without axons in the autonomous system which render the principle of one-directionality irrelevant. In this system, every stimulus immediately arouses the whole system. Perhaps this is the place to note that in the system of the skeletal muscles that are primarily connected with the central nervous system, there are fibers of the autonomous system and vice versa, fibers of the central nervous system are found in the whole autonomous system. Injury to the vegetative nerves influences standing tone, for example in the case of a very loud noise. There is also a connection between standing and the labyrinth system. This illustrates that the central and autonomous systems are not separate from one another and are meant to serve the individual together as one whole.

CHAPTER TWO
Potency and Movement

The organism's neuro-motor response has more energy than the stimulus that caused the response which means that the organism has stored potential energy. This energy is expressed in the response; the organism need not be occupied with creating energy when responding to the environment. Only once the activity is completed does the organism return to recharge its energy for potential future responses.

The abovementioned principle has survival value since it releases the organism from all other involvement while securing its safety and existence. The anti-gravitational tone also acts as a reflex, as we have already seen, and releases the animal from the need to be involved in all the extensive neuro-motor activities connected with standing in the gravitational field.

However, in contrast with anti-gravitational tone, which in principle is the contraction of the extensors, a mechanism connected to the fear of falling creates a subordinate pattern - that is to say – contraction of the flexors. In more developed animals, this mechanism also operates in other instances - an animal feels threatened when it is in the vicinity of an animal that it perceives as stronger. In the human being, anti-gravitational tone, which developed in evolution, reached its highest level in the animate world and enabled man to stand and walk on two feet. This erect posture provided several advantages to man for a more flexible and varied response to his environment.

a. The "moment of inertia" in this position is smaller than it is for other animals, meaning that less energy is required to create movement. This also enables a long distance walk.
b. The gravitational center is higher which means that there is more potential energy.
c. There is a possibility of a quicker and more effective response to stimulus from any direction.

It is worthwhile noting that one of the basic laws operating in the human being's neuro-motor system is that the level of differentiation is in reverse proportion to the amount of work that is done. For example, if someone places a ten-gram weight in our palm and adds another gram or two, we will feel the difference, but if someone places a one-kilo weight and adds a gram of two, we will be unable to tell the difference. In erect posture, the amount of work performed for standing and walking is minimal, and thus the person's level of differentiation in this posture is maximal (I will discuss this later). The higher the level of differentiation the greater the possibility of a more differentiated response to stimuli from the environment. This refers to kinesthetic stimuli; if the level of differentiation is higher, then a person can conduct himself more effectively in the gravitational field. In animals, the anti-gravitational tone activates the animal interactively, but in man, this tone which has evolved may possibly contradict the search for "security" in man's perception of himself in society. This will be expressed in the contraction of the flexors while anti-gravitational tone requires contraction of the extensors antagonistic to the flexors.

The live cell is the embodiment of dynamic balance in relation to the environment while in the human being, this balance was achieved in evolution, in the form of standing on two feet and carrying great mass in the upper part of the body (head and shoulders). An explanation of the concept of "effort" as opposed, perhaps, to the concept of work is appropriate here.

The concept of work is well-defined in the natural sciences and is ultimately connected to the movement of masses in the gravitational field. Effort can be defined as the condition in which more than necessary work is invested in order to perform a specific activity. On the surface, this seems irrational; why would a person invest more work than necessary? Below we will see the importance of the concept of "effort" and its connection to learning and creativity. When the rules of interactivity and solidarity function, there is no effort because the neuro-motor system is constructed to adjust the different parts in order to reach its goal.

Man, due to evolution, stands upright on both feet which provides more potential energy and at the same time, the possibility of responding with movement with minimal effort in every direction. Thus this upright state is the state of dynamic balance. The live cell is the embodiment of dynamic balance and in general, the animate is characterized as a state of potential energy, and movement with erect posture a heightened level of expression of both characteristics. The human being also has a psychic reality that lets him perceive himself as an object. This may cause his functioning to stem not from interactivity and solidarity but from a position that opposes the potential in erect posture.

On the one hand, the world of concepts facilitated man's high level of artistic and intellectual achievement and on the other, it facilitated pathological states. On the one hand, a word is meant to reflect organic authentic reality and on the other, a sterile intellectual world and in extreme examples, detachment from the experiential world.

CHAPTER THREE
Psychic Integration and the Concept of Mind

The concept of psychic integration connects with the concept of meaning. Paintings are sometimes open to different interpretations; what appears to be stairs in a painting may also be interpreted as an accordion. Interestingly, the mind becomes one when in a period of time it only gives a single meaning to the received stimulus. Clearly, psychic integration cannot be solely explained by the nervous system.

An additional characteristic of the mind is that consciousness is not engaged with what it cannot be effective in. There is extensive neuromotor activity after swallowing food, but consciousness is not involved in this activity and actually knows nothing about it. To generalize as I did in the introduction, the mind doesn't know how the neuromotor system works but can activate it for realizing a goal in the outside world; although I do not know how I stand, I do know that it is **I** who am standing. In the mind, control over the act and awareness of the act meet, I know that is I who am standing and I feel in control of the standing of my body in the gravitational field. The unification of the experience of this moment and this encounter is the **finite** mind.

As we will see later on, this feeling of self becomes vague in certain states and sometimes even totally disappears.

The two characteristics of integration and effectiveness (or economy) mentioned above are in accord since the moment the mind is not involved in the vegetative activity of digestion, it is available for providing meaning for additional external stimuli; this is essential, since its relationship with the outside impacts its ability to survive and protect itself.

Another important matter is the connection between the concept of mind and the concept of "subjective" time in contrast with "objective" time whose whole existence is in the comparison of different relative movements.

From the moment any organism makes any movements (in the sense of locomotion) to satisfy itself, from this moment the concept of mind begins to be formed (plants, an important part of the live world, do not have a mind).

The laws of physics – predicting beforehand what will happen - do not actually facilitate anything new happening. In evolution, in contrast, the appearance of a new type is also rooted in precise reasons, which means that if, after the fact, we knew the details of these reasons, we could explain the form that was created, the attempt to predict beforehand would come to nothing (Henri Bergson).

The behavior of the animate world differs from the inanimate world in two fundamental ways:
a. In animate activity, a process is moving towards a final cause.
b. One can never predict beforehand what will happen in this moving towards the cause. The animal stands to hunt its prey, works to realize this goal, but there is no way of knowing beforehand what will happen during these attempts. Time will be created in a different way than in the natural sciences, time whose extension causes the formation of something that did not exist beforehand that could also not have been predicted beforehand.

And behold, maybe we can begin to understand the connection between the concept of mind and the concept of time.

According to Sherrington, the information that enters through our two eyes does not unify spatially in our brain. Each eye receives a separate (and somewhat different) picture of the reality created when the rays of light fall on the retina and the nerve pulses (which are electric in their essence) reach the vision center of the brain.

Nonetheless, the mind recognizes that it is observing **one** reality because the observed event **happened in one specific period of time. Thus, time is the unifier of the mind.** The mind is also created in that I perceive all the different information that enters through my different senses as representing the same reality because with cooperation of all the senses and through movement I succeed in reaching my goal. On the other hand, the foundation of the mind that is movement towards realization of satisfaction, creates "subjective time" in the sense that there is an occurrence moving towards a final goal. We again clarify that in "objective" time nothing happens, only a specific object changed its place in relation to another object and this was pre-determined. In "subjective time", something happens that is not only measured in the two points t0..t1, but in what is between them, in the essence that is created which cannot be predicted beforehand and can only be "explained" afterwards.

We will see the profound significance of all this in everything relevant to learning and the art of performance.

As we have seen, "mind" takes on only one meaning in every period of time, but is also capable of doing only one **primary thing** in a period of time. This is something done on a different level of cognition than other things done at the same time, **which have the element of intention.** For example, when I write these words, I am occupied with the intention of clarifying and transmitting specific content but many other activities are happening simultaneously, such as my hand and body movements and bowel movements. These activities serve my intention (this is not always true) but they are not my intention and are on a lower level of cognition. We will see how this rule is disturbed and sometimes becomes very jumbled (this trait will be called "primary thing") in different interferences and neurotic performance.

This trait (**primary thing**) also helps the mind's primary task, which is the swift and precise organization on the time-space level, which is vital for continued existence, since there would be chaos if everything done at the same time were on the same level of cognition. In the mind – as we have seen – control of the action and awareness of the action meet. There is preparation for a mental goal and simultaneously performance of a coordinated movement of the muscles. In this context, the experience of pain is necessary despite the protective reflex. The reflex is seemingly sufficient but it only takes care of the injured part, while in pain, there is an integration of experience and knowledge that causes the action, for example, of going to the doctor. It is interesting to note in this context that when a person realizes that pain is not serving a protective purpose, he can ascribe another interpretation to pain that does not involve an action for the cessation of pain - for example, Moslems or Indians or masochists who afflict themselves with different tortures.

The mind speaks to us in the language of movement, just as nature speaks to us in the language of energy. Interestingly, the expansion of the mind in vertebrates was not primarily as a result of an addition of receptors or effectors, but because of more hierarchies in the brain that can activate the same muscles, that is to say, one can perform more intentions and the unity of the mind is created from a greater multiplicity. In man, most of the directionality functions are in the brain stem, but the eyes and consciousness also have control of these functions.

There are, for example, pathological states in which the patient cannot lift his hand when asked to do so, but can lift his hand when he wants to point to something interesting that he has seen. **The ability to realize different intentions in the same limbs reaches its highest level in man.**

The infant's awareness is shaped by his coordinated use of the skeletal muscles and teleceptors in order to realize his intentions. Gradually the movement becomes more conscious and voluntary in the sense of cause and effect in time and space. Intriguingly, the movement "itself" creates the awareness and afterwards becomes a conscious experience in the framework of awareness. Another somewhat related topic - I write with the help of my hand, **my hand does a specific activity but it is I who write, totally I.** This is the asymmetric quality of the mind. In fact, the development of the mind was made possible because the whole organism acted in accordance with its teleceptors. This follows the same principle, that the eyes or the ears lead the whole organism. The teleceptors introduce the concept of meaning into the system by giving increased power to the external stimuli and a breakthrough of advance actions that are geared to a conclusive final intention. If so, the concept of meaning is connected with the possibility of discerning whether preliminary actions serve or do not serve a conclusive intention. Therefore, a word will have specific meaning in a sentence spoken with a specific final intention. Later, I will discuss the question of building a verbal sentence and its connection to meaning. In the coordinated use of the different teleceptors and the skeletal muscles, one has the option of choosing in the present from past data towards a conclusive future cause as well as the possibility of recognizing the whole by a part that is the basis for the existence of the world of concepts. If, for example, an animal had many eyes, there would be chaos and the animal could not function as one organism. The animal's two eyes heighten the possibility of a more precise determination of objects in space, depth perception and increased resolution because of the overlapping of the two eyes.

The individual perceives all entering information as representing the same reality since when the different organs are coordinated, he succeeds in reaching his final goal. Thus the development of the mind is connected with the different sense organs and the element of movement. If someone, for instance, touches my hand in affection, then the mind is interested in dealing with it alertly, involved in what emphasizes someone else's solidarity with me and consequently my solidarity with myself as well. **Someone is just touching my hand but he is flooding my entire being with the feeling of solidarity.** A developed animal can also discern when someone touches his head in affection or aggression and is accordingly prepared as a whole entity.

Here, perhaps, it is worthwhile to mention the difference between perception and sensation. Perception means that the information from the external world reached my brain. This information has no meaning until the individual discovers the possibility of a relationship to this information. For example, when I see a triangle and I know and recognize a triangle in front of me, I then can point to it, draw it with my finger to show its angles and its place in space, lift it and so on. If in this moment of perception, all the components of a possible activity or response would be omitted, then this perception would be insignificant and not even reach consciousness. Sensation is integration of the mind in the face of a stimulus of the nervous system that occurs when we are interested in **what happens to our body at the specific moment and not the external event that occurs**. Consequently, the body image and its relationship to space are determining factors in every sensation and thus, in every conception. In mind, if so, there is also an encounter between a possible response and consciousness and some define the mind as the field of possible responses. The difference between differentiation and lack of differentiation is whether or not there is or is not a potential response ready for release in the form of a motor activity and the learning is actually the expansion of the boundary of behavior in relation to the objects. Interestingly, Freud defined trauma as a state of emotional pressure in which the individual does not have the outlet of a motor response, and hysteria – as a false type of motor expression to trauma.

The attempt to wield emotional pressure while teaching a child cannot achieve the appropriate motor responses and therefore cannot define sensations and conceptions for the child. Bergson and Dewey described man when he began to hunt as someone who was unable to hunt and had a vague perception of reality, since he did not have the appropriate motor responses and his intention of hunting contradicted his habitual responses, that is to say, an immutable holding of his eyes and hands.

An additional example is a child who peers through a microscope at tissue and sees something blurry and meaningless; however, when told what to expect, he then sees the tissue. This intention helps the child create a possible response to the object under the microscope, facilitating this recognition.

Chapter Three

Bertrand Russell explains the difference in how a thermometer and a human being feel cold. The thermometer measures a low temperature, but, in contrast with a human being, cannot say it knows that it is now cold, because it does not formulate a possible response to the cold. The thermometer does not wear a coat to warm itself.

Let us review and reiterate that the ability to recognize an object means the ability to find possible motor responses. These responses are a result of experience with organized action in the time-space dimension. But organized action means interactivity based on asymmetry. After many experiences of responses, which are expressed in movements, in relation to the information that enters through the teleceptors and especially the eyes, the objects become clear in our perception as such. From here we can perhaps understand why a word that serves as an all-inclusive representative of objects (the word "chair", for example, relates to all possible chairs) cannot be created in the mind before the sensory-motor processes occur. A close connection exists between action and meaning and there are those who define mind as a comprehensive field of possible meanings.

If words do not relate to potential action, they lose their ability to serve as language; this detachment occurs in pathological states. In World War I, when the wounded patients' afferent nerve ends were cut, they began to speak in meaningless sentences.

The unity of the mind is connected with the unification of the external object. The skier who has control of the ski slope "possesses the slope" and makes it a meaningful unit for himself.

However, our ability to differentiate is connected with something even more basic - awareness of our position and orientation in space. We cannot recognize without determining our position in space since we cannot respond to the external stimuli without these parameters. In this instance, the signals will be dull, distorted and meaningless, as sometimes happens when a person faints and doesn't immediately regain his orientation in space.

Reception of the pulses that come from the muscles to the brain is an important element in the existence of consciousness; in instances of the cessation of these pulses - if an animal's eyes were closed, it immediately sank into sleep; this is a state of very dull consciousness.

Since our perception of ourselves in space projects on our ability to create responses, this perception is also connected with the learning process that has at its core the ability to change our response according to our experience. But if it is difficult for us to formulate our own clear responses, it will be difficult to create clear experiences within ourselves, thus our self-perception in space and our ability to perform on the stage are connected.

Even the concept of causality is connected with guided and organized operation of the central nervous system that facilitates movement in time and space. In the responses of the vegetative system alone, one cannot find a connection between cause and effect.

Bertrand Russell claims that knowledge means acting correctly or acting appropriately. The movement towards achieving satisfaction, through organized activation of the sensors and effectors, created the possibility of signs; from the moment they were created, one could follow the distinction/separation between objective and subjective and between knowledge and error.

The peak of mind is creating a symbolic world that, on one hand, enables greater control and more discerning action, and on the other, lets the person see his body as an object that in pathological instances becomes foreign to him. Interactive-solidarity must exist not only in the organism but in the whole psycho-physical entity.

CHAPTER FOUR
Learning and Experiencing

Can one teach an infant to sit, stand, walk and speak? What does this question mean? To teach the infant these activities and for him to achieve mastery, one must know which muscles are used and in what sequence they must be activated to be performed; if, for instance, we are talking about sitting with different positions of the pelvis, back and head, then, to facilitate these variations of sitting, we would have to teach an infinite number of different uses of the different muscles in different ways.

This is impossible since we do not know the timing, which muscles to activate and the endless and different instructions necessary for all the possibilities. However, even if everything was known and possible, the infant still does not know how to follow and perform these instructions because he does not differentiate the different muscles, for say, sitting, as separate and distinct from one another (assuming that one could communicate with the infant).

Actually, when an adult wants to realize his intention, he doesn't know anything about his muscles' activity and doesn't experience the muscle contractions from within. He has the experience and the knowledge that he wants to do something (for instance, stand) and he is in control of his own standing.

We have already seen that there is an encounter between consciousness and control in the mind. This characteristic exists in potential and is implemented through experimentation. The baby makes different and varied movements from the day he is born and "suddenly", in a certain moment, he sits or stands etc. Several interesting components in this learning process can be observed:

a. Most of the activities for the purpose of learning to sit or stand are not attempts to sit or stand. The infant trains himself by implementing the different and varied movements that do not seem in any way connected to sitting or standing. This process is similar to the development of the live cell; although there is no miniature version of the physical characteristics - neither hair color nor hand shape - a person with a distinctive hand shape and specific hair color is created.

There is something in these primal elements that is not the thing itself and yet generates it.

b. The infant does not have advance conscious knowledge of the goal towards which he is heading, that is to say, sitting or standing etc. He does not know these concepts and it is doubtful that his world contains any concepts at all. The infant engages in actions towards the realization of something that he does not know about beforehand. Also, there is no involvement of consciousness in the sense that the infant says to himself, "Now you have to do this or that so that you can reach this or the other goal."

c. The actions that are done for learning sitting, standing etc, are varied and involve the whole neuro-motor system.

d. If the infant was not nudged too early on by people and was also not overprotected, then gravity was his primary teacher in the learning process. Gravity has two interesting characteristics as a teacher, one is consistency and two, there is no emotional pressure in the learning process.

e. The infant performs most of his actions on his own initiative. And he is tireless in continuing with them despite his lack of success and the blows that he absorbs.

f. There is an adjustment process between means and goals that does not stem from irrelevant considerations.

Perhaps we can conclude from the above, that the learning process is inherent in the infant as an inborn need and ability. If the infant does not do the actual learning himself, no one can do it for him. This is similar to the infant's process of development into a child. If he on his own doesn't become a child, nothing in the world can make this happen.

There is a similarity between the infant's learning process and the processes which began in evolution, when man underwent the process of becoming upright and standing on his two feet. We have already seen the advantages of standing upright in the chapter "Potency and Movement". From the force of evolution, the infant has the desire and ability to learn to stand straight and be in a more potent state than lying or walking on four. There is potential energy in standing. That is to say, the learning process leads to a more potent state than what existed before.

We assume that the same traits that characterize the animate world of interactivity and solidarity with oneself are also inherent in the infant and that the infant teaches himself without violating or distorting these traits. All this on the condition that he was not nudged and overly pressured to do activities too-early and that he was not overprotected.

The animal's same ability to perform organized activities in the right order within the dimension of time is connected to inherent inhibited reflexes and processes, while the human being has a quite long and complex training period. Through experience and knowledge of the environment, processes of inhibition are created which facilitate the creation of ordered activities in the dimension of time. No one can teach the infant to inhibit the activation of this neuron or to activate another neuron in a given period of time and the infant himself (like the adult) does not experience any inhibition or activation in his brain activity.

Learning, if so, is connected to processes of inhibition that do not reach consciousness and therefore, at its core, is not a conscious process. It is latent and based on an inherent trait of inhibition connected to experience. The function of the central nervous system is not behavior but doing one primary thing in a period of time when the rest of the elements are inhibited. If its function were behavior, then there would be chaos due to the diffuse activation.

In the process of learning to ride a bicycle, for example, many of the movements are first done diffusely; the organization of orderly movements in the dimension of time comes gradually. From the moment that the skill is successfully acquired, involvement with the details sinks to the unconscious which then leaves room for innovativeness in the bike riding experience, such as the riding of acrobats in the circus.

Forming each letter demands the young child's entire attention; in contrast, the attention of the mature person who has successfully learned to write is not directed to how his fingers form the letters, but to the thoughts that the words express.

In development and in the learning process, there is also a gradual transition from responses to polymorphous sensations, connected primarily with the vegetative system, to responses connected with the individual's response as a whole to one limb, for example, eyes or ears etc. This response is made with the skeletal muscles that are connected to the cortex via the pyramid track together with the teleceptors which are also connected there.

It is interesting to note in this context that Freud claimed that in sexual development, there is a transition from amorphous sexual feelings to the feeling that sexuality is primarily centered on one organ (the sexual organ).

In the successful learning process, higher (cortical) hierarchies enter which facilitate a more refined and elaborate response. Inhibitions are formed that make possible gradation and moderation in response without violating the student's interactivity and solidarity.

The result of the successful learning process is the right division of labor coordinated between the different muscles that carry and move the body in the gravitational field; some view this division of labor as a sign of mental health.

The infant builds his **consciousness** together with the process in which he learns to walk, stand, etc.- a process in which there is interaction in the cortex between the system of neurons that activate the skeletal muscles in voluntary activity and the neurons that are connected to the teleceptors. Therefore, when blindness strikes, for example, at a young age, all the functions connected with vision are destroyed, but if blindness occurs in adulthood, then the sensations of visual direction, visual memory and the standing reflexes are retained.

We have seen that at a young age all information that enters through the teleceptors represents a sensory-motor and vegetative disturbance. We have also seen that standing and walking are the result of a process in which the skeletal muscles and the teleceptors participate. This is the source of the dynamic meaning of the term "posture" which means how a person carries himself, moves and perceives himself. He uses himself in the way that he perceives himself and this perception connects to the process in which he learned to walk, stand and so on. Therefore, how this posture was achieved is most important as well as whether or not there is a contradiction between how he uses his body and his state of mind. Instead of reflexive responses common to mankind that activate the individual in an undiscerning and sweeping fashion, control and awareness are gradually created in the learning process which facilitate deconstructing the past into its elements, so that one can choose what is appropriate to the current situation. In evolution and also in the ascending ladder of levels of life, there are, as we have said, more "masters" to the same "servants" (effectors) that provide more of an opportunity for different intentions. In his development, the infant builds within himself these "masters" until he reaches the level in which he can perform in any period of time, one primary activity which is on a higher cognitive level than the other activities and with an element of intention.

This is, perhaps, the place to discuss the question of intention and the sensation of free will. Seemingly, all the deterministic rules apply to the brain as a physical-chemical entity of the natural sciences and accordingly every state of mind at T1 totally and absolutely depends on the state of mind at T0, that is to say, there is no possibility of free choice. Whatever happens in the future depends absolutely and totally on what happened in the past.

However, in my opinion, the feeling of free will could be connected with the concept of understanding. We have stated that the goal of science is to deconstruct the whole into its parts so that the relationship of the parts with one another and with the whole is revealed. When there is interactivity and the asymmetric quality and the trait of "primary action" on the higher cognitive level with the element of intention, then there is a feeling of free will, "free" in the sense that one feels like continuing the activity, **continuing to realize the intention which is clarified with its actualization,** without any feeling of internal opposition to doing or a sense of dullness. The infant in training himself to walk, sit and stand continues on and on in his actions, despite the difficulties that he encounters. When I teach myself to play J.S. Bach's *Partite* on the piano and my hands, eyes and ears and all the neuro-motor system together serve the intention of expressing, deepening and understanding the music more and more, I have a feeling of free will. There is no internal opposition to this process of searching and clarification and I feel the need to continue with my playing on and on. Here, as in science, there is a sensation of discovering the relationship between the parts and the whole while in this instant the whole is the **finite** mind that is created in every moment that I play with the different parts in total harmony. It is my finger that touches the keyboard but I am wholly absorbed in the process of expression and search and emotion.

One can summarize and say that the feeling of free will is connected with the need to build the finite mind. The need to find the potential encounter of control, knowledge and experience or intention in the activity that I do, of creating something new that could not be predicted beforehand.

Possibly our task as educators and teachers is to have the student experience how his own diverse faculties serve the trend of potency, or in other words, of a richer and more whole **finite** mind. We must reemphasize that we are not talking about appealing to the student's consciousness or encouraging will by emotional pressure connected to these or other values, but perception of the student as of ultimate value with the whole purpose of learning intended to help him more fully realize his potential. Conscious dictation of values and the creation of a "strong will" may be in deep internal contradiction to the experiential reality and create pressure and even a breakdown. See Deborah Kobobi's book (Therapeutic Teaching). There are many difficult questions on building the child's world of concepts that do not always go hand in hand with our intuition and common sense (for example, dividing a fraction by a fraction).

Interestingly, in physics, analysis of the homogeneity in nature brought us to the level of abstraction. It seems to me that one can adopt a similar approach to the learning process and the student's entry into the conceptual world. One should analyze the student according to the different components of mind (see the chapter on psychic integration and the concept of mind) and insure that the transition to the world of concepts does not destroy his homogeneity in his perception of the world and of self.

What is the meaning of homogeneity?

The natural sciences have taught us that all the observed phenomena in the material world are of one kind; they represent one world and not different worlds. The idea of belief in one God, and not worshipping different gods who sometimes fight with each other, seems important in the context of a homogeneous *weltanschaung* and is an expression of the person's drive to discover one world for himself and thus unify himself.

The child will perceive the unified reality around him by amassing discerning responses that connect with his self-activation in interactivity and solidarity while preserving and developing the basic traits of the mind. The process of building and uniting the mind will occur together with the perception of the reality around him as one reality, since the child will be able to act in his environment and find satisfaction as **one whole entity**. His feeling that he can act as a whole entity in relation to his environment will cause the perception that unifies the reality.

We have seen that the child has the characteristic traits of the animate world, interactivity and solidarity, and the potential of mind based on the principles discussed. It seems to me that if in the child's different experiences, these traits and principles are not assaulted or violated, he will have a homogeneous *weltanschaung* and consequently the experience of uniting himself vis-à-vis the objects and their perception as such (as concepts).

We have seen that the mind can be the seat of only one meaning in one period of time and this trait is inherent in potential in the infant from birth (if this were not so, it would be impossible to teach him that there is any meaning to the hodgepodge of information that enters his brain). This again illustrates that the ability to organize and conceptualize reality is inherent from birth. If the learner uses the asymmetric principle correctly while preserving interactivity and solidarity, then the meanings will pop up by themselves and the foundation for the conceptual world will be set. To give **only one** specific meaning to the entering information and utilize the surrounding objects asymmetrically and interactively means to build concepts within ourselves. Unifying the objects around us and their perception as such and the unifying of the brain minute-by-minute (the finite mind) are inborn needs that originate in evolution. The abstraction is, then, the process of generalization through action.

Chapter Four

One can perhaps compare the law of preserving energy in nature with the law of preserving the finite mind as something one and whole. It seems to me that it would be correct to say that even in neurotic and psychotic states, the aspiration and need to fulfill this law causes pathological phenomena. (I will discuss this in the chapter on the State of Disorder).

Building the intellectual world seems to depend on sensory-motor functions that accumulate with experience. Experience accumulates in two forms:
a. Motor mechanisms
b. Memory of body image

Thus nature stores information authentically and memory is articulated in the total action.

It is true, indeed, that a word should help deconstruct past experience and thus facilitate behavior according to the present circumstances, but this on condition that it was hewn from the organic, otherwise it may be an empty vessel that does not represent language in the sense of relationship to environment and self.

The pulses that reach our brain from the muscles are of utmost importance and only information about pain is more important. Unfortunately, these pulses do not reach our consciousness and our motor responses and positions sink into the unconscious with the passing of time. The pain pushes me to go to the appropriate doctor, but what can be done with the valuable information that I am unaware of and which nonetheless supplies the necessary background for the meaning of the information that reaches me through my environment, since it is the storehouse of my authentic memory. All the meanings are connected to this background but it does not reach consciousness and cannot be conceptualized. Here, there is no principle of consciousness and control that exists in the mind and causes me to know that it is **I** who am standing and feel control over my standing; as we have seen, **I do not have knowledge and I do not have control of how I interpret and explain my environment.** We have seen that self-awareness is constructed in a sensory-motor process and within that framework the child teaches himself to sit, walk and stand; we have seen that every sensory disturbance at a young age is a vegetative sensory-motor disturbance.

My comprehension of the environment and the objects (including myself) is interwoven in a way that cannot be separated from earlier experiences, which are the true storehouse of my memory - for example, from the time that I learned the word "mother" connected to a specific woman who stimulated a specific sensory-motor response, it is impossible to cancel the accumulation of memory connected to the word "mother".

The question arises when relating to a word - how can it be connected with loaded material that I really do not know. Words have an all-encompassing nature; for example, the word "chair" relates to all possible chairs.

A word has the advantage of encoding many different and heterogeneous objects into one concept which makes it easier to transmit "objective" information, but the word "chair" does not relate to any specific chair in its uniqueness. In certain circumstances the word may blur the experience until there is absolute detachment, it may detach the topic of "sitting" (in connection with the word chair) from all content and leave it sterile without the vitality of life. This is a type of response that fits many situations, **but not any specific situation**, therefore a word has meaning if it arouses an organic response.

Clearly, the concept formation has survival value for mankind, since it facilitates more precise planning for the future. We have also seen that the ability of abstraction is connected to orderly action in the time-space level. When there is too-early emotional pressure, appeal to consciousness and detachment from experiencing, a pathetic world of concepts may be formed that the person clutches as a lifesaver when roaming the depths of the experiential world.

This is a caricature of mind that does not fulfill the basic principle of unity in multiplicity and cannot, by its very nature, fulfill the other principles latent in the animate and in the mind.

Another worthwhile discussion in the topic of experiencing and learning are matters of time. One can innumerate several types of time; we have seen how time unifies the mind and how the building of the mind, which at its core is movement to actualize satisfaction, creates time in the sense of occurrence moving towards a goal.

The inferior creature in the early stage of evolution was actually a slave to happenstance. Without teleceptors and brain ganglions it could not "predict" the future in the sense of interactive organization towards fulfilling a goal in the future. The infant is also only a slave to primarily vegetative pulses, which determine sleeping and waking hours. In adapting to the gravitational field, using the skeletal muscles and teleceptors, he builds his own sense of "subjective" time connected to his organization towards realization of intentions.

An advantage of "objective" time is that the homogeneity enables us to remember dates and places. In the healthy development process, a coordinated and flexible integration develops between these two times, and "behavior time" is created. In extreme examples of unhealthy development, the phenomenon of a "continuous present" may sometimes develop in the psychotic, or in the neurotic, the phenomena of self-effacement and hysterical behavior regarding objective time.

The topic of time is central to learning processes and to creating a character in the theater. These processes should preferably be done "**in the rhythm of rest,**" that is to say, without a demand for too-early results. This demand may violate the elements of interactivity and solidarity and connect the actual learning process to the state in which the human being loses his ability to regulate his own well-being. I will discuss this important question further.

When the infant learns with adult assistance, he is unaware of how the adult guides him and he cannot create his own alternatives. The infant practices towards sitting and walking at his own pace, coordinating all the different faculties.

In educating children it is terrible to plant the belief that a specific self-use threatens them. This is a sure recipe for weakening ability and self-perception and in extreme cases may cause a break in the individual's organic and psychic reality. The psychotic who does not perceive his bodily pain as his own has actually detached his psychic reality from his organic reality; perhaps this detachment provided a sense of security when he was under great emotional pressure and had no other available alternatives.

There are those who claim that the brain operates according to what the "owner of the brain" believes; it seems to me that an experiment was even conducted which proved that the optic center responds to different light intensities according to the beliefs of the "owner of the brain" and not according to the physical intensity that was radiated.

We repeat that in early childhood every experience which is connected, for example, with the teleceptors, there is always a sensomotoric-vegetative disturbance. I remember that the first time I left Jerusalem as a child to go hiking in the green areas of the lowlands, I saw a color green that I have never again had the privilege of seeing in later periods of my life.

The attempt to help the child build a world of concepts should not narrow his experiential world, which is nothing but the same senso-motoric disturbance. When my daughter was a three and four year old, her paintings were rich and bold and one could even discern the element of composition in the sense of unity within multiplicity. And then came first grade and everything was erased as though it never existed. Her "orderly" paintings were dull and detached from any experiences. Nothing in them was reminiscent of a developing process of creativity.

Something in her organic ability to express was destroyed, perhaps irreparably. There was a detachment between the **concept** of house that she tried to draw according to the teacher's expectations and her own organic experience of this concept.

The discernment and the sensomotoric-vegetative disturbance were essentially the same thing. We have already seen that knowing is identical with discerning (someone looking into a microscope) but if we prevent the varied and comprehensive neuro-motor response, we impoverish and blur the experience and consequently the knowing. The knowing in this instance will resemble trying to remember words in a foreign language without its wide and deep foundation, without the associations to arouse feeling (other, perhaps, than the feeling of foreignness), without the sense that the specific word was chosen from many different options in the individual's rich inner world.

We have seen that accumulated experience is also connected with the memory of the self-image. If education in early childhood narrowed or negated this image, then the mature adult can only use himself in a limited fashion and every attempt to extricate himself from these chains will be difficult and unlikely to succeed.

Skills are not only a repetition of set actions, they also have innovativeness and progress. One doesn't repeat the same movements in exactly the same ways. However in skills, there must be an element of consistency and stability in time and space, which must not replace the opportunity for change and learning through doing. A performance does not only mean movement in relation to discreet components, one at a time. One can distinguish a "structure" concealed in movements using information on the timing of the serial movements and the "mistaken patterns" that occur in the performing of the series of movements. This same "structure" is connected, in my opinion, with the memory of body image which makes me utilize myself in one way and not another. Body image is connected with how the organism moves and operates as an entity in the gravitational field and social environment. Thus, if we want to repair things we must also treat the psycho-motor question of the body moving in the gravitational field. I learned from experience how very differently man uses himself if he is acting under the title of teacher or student or friend, etc. How much a person uses himself returns to interactivity-solidarity when someone else is willing to be an enthusiastic address for his actions.

Chapter Four

In developed animals the asymmetric trait exists, especially in the passive sense of the word. The whole body, the whole animal responds to the information that enters, for instance, through the eyes. Although this trait also exists in the active sense when the animal is using its claws to catch its prey, these two examples are different. In the first example, **there is purposeful walking towards a future goal.** The animal sees its prey and its whole body moves towards it, but in active use **there is only the current action. Active asymmetric action which points towards a future goal can also be considered as the beginning of language in the human sense.**

The possibility of actively implementing the asymmetric trait in the future also facilitates the distinction between myself and the other and therefore facilitates a conscious relationship to myself. It is **I** who points with **my** hand towards a possible future goal.

The animal is totally absorbed in its immediate survival needs when it grasps its prey in its two front claws. Learning must not cause man to be totally absorbed in doing without the ability for innovativeness and change.

We have already seen that this is a characteristic of skills with the potential for innovativeness. Bergson illustrates this with an example of two different people who operate the same machine. One person is totally absorbed in the machine while the other person operates the machine, attentive to self and to the environment. The first person will be unable to innovate or improve anything in the machine and in the production process while the second person may be able to discover new things, innovate and invent. The artificial attempt to "concentrate" may result in superficial and shallow action which leaves no room for creativity.

Speech is, it seems to me, the apex of the active asymmetric trait because the principle of unification of man exists in the sense of idea-feeling-self perception – relationship to the environment while using the vocal mechanism.

Learning is a process in which something foreign gradually becomes ingrained. At first I have to discover how something is an option for me, then I have to find a comfortable way to make it happen and then how it will be enjoyable to do so. A successful process requires a discerning eye that examines all the components of the student, each separately and the whole together (the student). Assimilation occurs when I know how to do what I have learned by interactivity and solidarity action. Successful learning does not violate the principle of unity in multiplicity but enriches it by discovering additional and varied connections between the different faculties.

One must pay special attention to the moment the specific system of responses is abandoned and no other clear system is yet built. This is the dangerous moment in the entire process and if not done delicately and with the teacher's attentive listening, there may be regression or a pathetic hanging on to the blurry knowledge, like a person clutching a straw.

In summation, we must ask ourselves if education in the school system doesn't destroy interactivity and solidarity. Do we enable the student to advance at his own rhythm to the satisfying goal of building his mind? Are we disruptive of his intentions? The learning process is going towards the unknown while creating responses along the way that were unknown beforehand. In a successful process, there is a sense of choosing the means in order to realize the goals; in this process the goals also become clearer.

The blurring of intentions, which is the blurring of the body image and the mind, is connected to the "intention" of appeasing the teacher. The student who feels unsafe and unsure in not fulfilling the teacher's expectations may destroy his ability for potent action and lose the ability to learn while preserving his well-being. The inborn traits of interactivity and solidarity and the inborn characteristics of the mind may be confused forever.

Animals that were placed in a cage who received everything they were lacking in food and sex, responded negatively to this situation. They were lacking all the **behaviors** associated with searching for their own gratification. This very process of building their own mind seems to have been lacking.

CHAPTER FIVE
A State of Disorder

The response to threat is inherent not only in man but in the entire developed animate world. The response includes, among other things, muscle contraction and accelerated activity of the heart and diaphragm. This response has survival value since it prepares the organism for the possibility of fight or flight. The flexors that contract first (their response is faster) facilitate more intensive activity in the next phase, of the extensors, which were inhibited, for fight or flight.

The accelerated activity of the heart and the diaphragm brings a greater supply of oxygen to the brain and muscles and makes possible vigorous activity to remove the threat. When the animal attacks or escapes, it utilizes everything that was prepared in the organism; once the threat is removed, the animal returns to a state of homeostasis. The response to threat is reflexive (and therefore also stereotypical), sweeping and undifferentiated. It is intended to immediately guarantee the survival of the animal when there is insufficient time for a refined and elaborate response. In the state just described, the two parts of the autonomous nervous system operate and inhibit one another (antagonists). The sympathetic part prepares the animal for a response and the parasympathetic part returns to homeostasis and healing from the experienced trauma. The activity of the heart and the diaphragm is slowed down and the muscles return to their normal tone that is bound up with the animal's normal response to its environment – vigilance.

In more developed animals, physical confrontation is avoided by the "surrender" of the animal who perceives the other animal as stronger. In this state, the surrendering animal's head drops, it glances sideways and breathes irregularly. This behavior also has survival value as it prevents a physical struggle that could end with endangered life and loss.

It is appropriate to note here that after a brief training period, developed animals (with hooves and teleceptors) develop a potent anti-gravitational stance, enabling them to look at their environment as well as have rather efficient movement in the gravitational field. The head is in a position that lets the eyes be at a permanent angle relative to the perpendicular of the gravitational field. Even the chick hatched from the egg has an upright head so that its eyes turn forward and not downward (this has an element of potency, the possibility of control over the environment).

Man, as we have already said, has the potential for potent standing on two feet, but must first undergo a quite long training period. In fact, the infant undergoes a process of adaptation to gravity, a process that man apparently underwent for many years, in the process of evolution. Since the main function of the central nervous system, as we have seen, is to maintain and move the body in the gravitational field as one unit, we can perhaps learn about its functioning by how man carries and moves his body.

In successful adaptation to gravity, man will achieve a potent standing on his feet. It is true that human beings who grew up around other human beings learned to stand on their two feet but they did not all realize the potent options similarly. There is something stereotypic in how the animal holds and moves his body (the "animal" referred to lives in nature and is not under human control), while the human being has more ways of holding his body and walking in the gravitational field.

We have seen that the infant practices his own varied movements, which results in sitting, walking, standing and so on. It is true that the infant needs the company of people to achieve these results, but we have also seen that he cannot be taught how to achieve them and if he doesn't learn on his own, he will not acquire them.

This process of adaptation to gravity is unusually complex; instructions to a man-robot on how to sit, stand, and walk would be interlaced with many complex calculations and almost endless instructions, since there are endless different combinations.

We have seen that this process of adaptation to gravity also occurs in the process of the infant's building his consciousness and ability to discern cause and effect. With the building of the pyramid track in the cortex, different connections are formed between stimuli from the teleceptors and stimuli from the muscles and thus the opportunity of perceiving the objects as such is shaped.

The adaptation process is more complex in the hips and the neck (occiput), because of the following reasons:
a. In both the hips and the neck, circular movements can be made in relation to the environment.
b. The entire body weight rests on the lumbar area while quite precise directionality in relationship to the stimuli in the environment is simultaneously required.
c. The use of the teleceptors requires the precise and fast direction of the neck muscles to turn the head, which is relatively heavy, towards the location of the stimulus.

Chapter Five

The nervous system functions with its level of differentiation in inverse proportion to the amount of work performed. In the lumbar and neck, there must be great discernment although too much weight rests on them. This explains the complex and prolonged training necessary for maintaining the body perpendicular to the ground.

In successful learning, man will achieve potential uprightness with a minimal amount of work in the skeletal muscles and a well-distributed work distribution among the different muscles. We have seen that the same muscles are meant to receive "instructions" from different hierarchies in the brain, that is to say, there is a possibility of instructions contradicting one another. What characterizes potent standing is the fact that the skeletal system receives "instructions" that are not contradictory, which meshes with the interactivity of the neuro-motor system.

The possibility of disorder happens in two ways:
a. Under emotional pressure, the infant is expected to do things too-early
b. The infant is overprotected as an "incentive" in the learning process.

In the second instance, there is also some obtuseness since, on one hand, the infant is given incentives to advance and on the other, he is related to as someone who cannot advance. In both instances, the infant is asked to do something he does not yet know how to do. This demand comes with a threat to his security - if he doesn't do this he is likely to lose the love of the grown-ups on whom he depends for survival.

In the neuro-motor system, contradictory processes will be created. On one hand, the aspiration to potent learning inherent in the child from the power of evolution and on the other, defense in the face of the threat being made against him.

When there is overprotectiveness, the infant will sense that his potent use of his body in the learning process endangers his security, since the adults, by their overprotective behavior, broadcast that they want him to be someone who can't succeed and is helpless. "Noise" will be created in his nervous system that serves neither the need of protection nor the need of potency.

We have seen that the response to threat is impulsive and undifferentiated and connected with contracting the flexors while the aspiration to stand straight is connected with contracting the extensors which are the antagonists of the flexors. Ultimately the child will stand on his own feet but in a caricature of standing which does not send a clear message of potency and does not have all the characteristics of correct erect posture (see chapter Potency and Movement). The child will learn that learning and doing are connected to "effort" and a state of "noise".

Why effort? Since in the caricature of standing described above, more than necessary power is invested which is due the contracted flexors working against standing. The child will learn that in the learning process he loses his ability to regulate his own well-being. The quality of interactivity and solidarity will be distorted and consequently the feeling of the self in the learning process and in performance will be very blurry.

Let us review again where the feeling that it is **I** who is active stems from. We have seen that the basis of mind is in movement to achieve satisfaction and this movement is made with a coordination of the different parts, that is to say, movements that are coordinated in the time-space dimension and the solidarity of the whole with its parts. In contrast, failed learning has no satisfaction because it contains an implicit threat. There is no solidarity because the infant uses his body despite internal opposition to action, since the self is not yet ready for performance and there is no interactivity because there is no coordination and in actuality, there is contradiction within the neuro-motor system. The acquired knowledge is like clutching the final straw without the total involvement of the self and without the possibility of innovation because of the continuous and circular involvement in the question of the desire to achieve potency versus the deep feeling of inability. Innovativeness occurs when the skill is acquired in interactivity and solidarity that enables the details of the performance to sink into the unconscious without their disturbing the person with additional processes.

Anxiety can be defined as the state in which man believes that he has only one option. Just this and no other. We will illustrate with the example of a man who has to walk on a beam that is 20cm wide. The beam is not anxiety-producing when placed on the floor because the person knows that even if he falls off the beam nothing terrible will happen. If the beam is placed at a height of 5 meters, the person will be in a state of anxiety since he knows that he has only one option - to walk on the beam; if he cannot walk across he will endanger himself. However, the person's response to this threat will be contraction of flexors and the other responses that we have listed. This response will usually lead to failure since there is less possibility of control and of discriminating the relationship to the pulses from the environment (See the advantages of potent posture in the chapter on Potency and Movement).

In failed learning, specific conditioning occurs:
a. Learning is an unpleasant process connected with effort in which the self is not fully involved.
b. Doing is connected with a deep inner feeling of inability.
c. If he was overprotected then the will to implement something potent will produce anxiety and thwart the possibility for potent action.

In actuality, the learning process stops, in the sense of something that is gradually built based on the inborn traits of the animate and the mind. Every pathological state can be described as a state of stopping the learning process and getting stuck in circularity without a way out.

The literature talks about the positive connection between clear boundaries, perception of self-image and other variables. When boundaries are very clear, the goals and standards are clear, there is a strong desire to fulfill the task, confidence in the ability to achieve, better self-direction within the different alternatives and independence and the ability of assertive expression. It was also found that people with clear boundaries have more aspirations, that is the search for something higher, better and more refined.

People with unclear boundaries have confused concepts and a blurring of the principle of cause and effect. A connection between schizophrenic states and unclear boundaries has been discovered. It seems to me that the model that I have just presented can explain these connections in an immanent fashion. We have seen that in an unsuccessful process of learning the skills of standing, walking etc, two contradictory paths are created in the neuro-motor system and neuro-motor "noise" is created. We have also seen that the infant is meant to build his consciousness, that is to say, his consciousness of the environment as well as a distinctive self-awareness in the learning process. In a successful process, the teleceptors and the skeletal muscles are coordinated (both have cortical representation). The child learns that coordinated activation of his teleceptors and skeletal muscles will bring the hoped-for result, gratification of his needs. He constructs within himself the option of doing one primary thing on a higher cognitive level in a period of time with the element of intention which is possible when all the different faculties operate in mutual reinforcement to realize the goal. The clear boundary between my environment and myself is created when I take what I need for my satisfaction from the environment - I work with the environment **as one whole entity with one clear direction in a time frame** and thus I also have one clear internal message that my desire to negotiate with my environment does not harm my base as a living being, that is to say, my interactivity and my solidarity with myself. As we have already seen, the construction of concepts and the principle of cause and effect is connected with interactivity and solidarity and with building the characteristics of the mind based on it.

I claim that the child's clear boundaries are built in the process of acquiring skills, if the process occurred without too-early demand and without overprotectiveness. In a successful process all the other variables are created as well: clear goals, passion, confidence in the ability to achieve goals and so on. The infant does not stop training towards the goal and all his bruises do not discourage him or undermine his efforts, that is to say, they do not shake his confidence. We have seen that creating the world of concepts is connected with an orderly activity in the time-space dimension and the principle of cause and effect is formed by mutual reinforcement of different faculties in the path to achieving satisfaction. All this will be distorted if the trait of interactivity and solidarity is distorted. Aspirations will not be formulated if the skills were not acquired in interactivity and solidarity since there will be ongoing involvement with the unresolved details of performance.

There are those who claim that the psychotic sometimes perceives his body as not belonging to him. According to our proposed model, this happens when the contradictions are too great, when it is impossible to hold on to both sides, to continue in the "noise" of the inner contradiction. The psychotic who wants to preserve the "unity" of his mind will separate himself from his body. Even in killing himself the psychotic will not realize that he is destroying his being but, rather, thinks that he is freeing himself from the contradictions in his search for unity. Killing himself is the one thing that he can plan clearly, in terms of cause and effect. In situations of too-early demands and overprotectiveness, there is no clear goal. The child is unclear as to what his goal is - should he appease the adult or teach himself?

We have seen that unity of the mind is connected with unifying the meaning given to external stimuli. However, in this case, there is no chance of giving one meaning to these stimuli and no possibility of creating one orientation in a period of time. The stimuli from gravity connected with evolution do not correspond with the stimuli from adults, who demand a too-early result which is threatening.

Standing, in a state of "noise", the level of differentiation also decreases since the amount of work that is done is far greater than in a potent state. We have seen that the human being's nervous system is built so that the level of differentiation is in reverse proportion to the amount of power invested. Therefore it is not surprising that there is a connection between relying on kinesthetic signs and the ability to preserve spatial

Chapter Five

orientation in a mistaken state. People who relied more on these signs also demonstrated more body interaction and sexual maturity.

Someone who acquired the skills of standing and walking unsuccessfully reached standing with a low level of differentiation and is therefore less able to respond to the kinesthetic signs and in the same breath one can say that the unsuccessful process undermined the latent interactivity and ability to function as a whole according to one organ limb leading the whole being (the asymmetric principle). And this is sexual maturity, the ability to utilize my whole self in response to the stimulus to primarily one organ (sexual organ). The too-early demand also did not allow the child to experience mistakes in the learning process and find his own solutions. Consequently, he cannot remain oriented in a misleading situation as he was not given the opportunity to experience this, to create different responses to different and varied situations.

We have seen that consciousness does not get involved when it cannot be effective. In successful learning the acquired skills sink into the unconscious and consciousness is not involved with them and is available for other stimuli, both internal and external. However in an unsuccessful process, consciousness will be unnecessarily occupied with the details. For example, when there is a vague threat, consciousness will be involved with breathing, which usually is reflexive and according to need.

A sixty-year-old woman turned to me for help – because of her difficulty breathing when she exercises, she gets involved with the breathing process. To my question of why she exercises, she answered that people in the know told her that if she didn't exercise she would most probably fall apart. I asked her what exactly would happen if she didn't exercise? Her response was, "I don't know." At a certain moment, this woman became aware of her struggle with an unclear threat in these exercises. There was no possible interactive response and therefore, her awareness descended to "the details of the performance" - in this instance, breathing.

We have learned from the field of communications that when there is an unclear relationship with the other or my own self-perception towards the other is unclear or there is an attempt to hide something from the other, then awareness will "descend" to involvement with the details such as: How do I hold my hand? How do I speak? How does the other look at me?

The excellent actor or the superb philosopher is not involved with the doing of "actions" but is absorbed in a process of clarification. That is to say, something that was unclear beforehand is clarified. Usually, understanding occurs after the process, because as Bertrand Russell says, we do not understand our contemporary experience; it will only be able to be explained after the fact. In general, there is a danger in the learning process that because of emotional pressure and an unclear demand, the student will hold onto "the doing of actions" **involved in the action instead of the direction or intention.** In an improved state, there is a sensation of unity of intention and action, they are perceived as one; for the neurotic, this is not always the case. For example, if the described harmony doesn't exist when I write these lines, then I will find myself involved with the muscles of my fingers and hands and I will perceive my hand as foreign, as though it isn't wholly mine. The asymmetric principle will not exist, according to which my hand is involved with writing but it is I who is in the process and intention of clarifying something to myself and to the other.

Chapter Five

In my class at the Institute for Education in Jerusalem, I asked one of the students (in a course for teachers tracked to be school principals) to move her head in a specific way. After she had done this movement several times, it became clear from our conversation that there were two primary aspects to her movements:
a. She herself was not involved in the performance.
b. She wanted to make the movement perfectly and immediately.

Doesn't this sound familiar? This is the same issue as the failed learning process, in which there is no involvement of the self but, nonetheless, there is a demand for immediate and superior performance.

This woman, whom I tried to guide, apparently internalized this connection with the learning of something unknown and unclear - "I am not involved and yet I expect of myself to do it perfectly."

At the end of this class, the student had an improved understanding of the text (topic of the class) and felt more involved when she read the same chapter in the Bible. If so, one can see that there is a continuum in the range of different situations starting from an interactive-potent state up until a psychotic state. It is all just a question of the extent to which man's interactivity and psycho-physical solidarity were destroyed.

Psychosis (schizoid or depressive) can be described as the effort to unify the mind with imaging of a state in which the human being had control of the results. Longstanding involvement in the circularity of unresolved things can cause the person to invent "solutions" and "explanations" that don't solve or explain anything since there is a "vicious circle" of causes that are results and results that are causes.

It is interesting to note again that the schizophrenic sometimes has a state of "continuous present". This also seems to be in accord with the proposed model.

Let us remember for a moment the beginning of the creation of the subjective time dimension, when the animal moves toward its goal of satisfaction through mutual reinforcement of the different factors and through interactivity and solidarity. The schizophrenic's interactivity and solidarity is so destroyed that he cannot act as a whole unit toward realizing a future goal.

A fiftyish year-old man who came to me for problems with his voice was asked to lie on his side and bend his knee. This simple movement was difficult for him and it soon became apparent that he made muscular movements in his thigh and hip that prevented the knee-bending. He was in a state of "effort" (defined as the investment of more than necessary power towards the realization of a specific intention). Clearly the muscular movements which were antagonistic to the bending of the knee, made the bending difficult and perhaps impossible. I asked my student in the School for Acting to lie on his side and imagine the movement of bringing the knee close to the stomach area. I asked if he thought that when his knee made this movement, there would be movement in the thigh as well. His answer was, "Of course," since the thigh is connected to the knee and every movement of the knee must necessarily pull along the movement of the thigh. It became apparent that in his visualization there was an imaginary movement of the knee without an imaginary movement in the thigh. **The thigh "refused" to adapt itself to the movement in the knee.**

This was not surprising as it corresponded with our non–interactive use of ourselves in the whole process of learning something new.

Indeed, the effort is the agent that dictates the continued use that we make of ourselves that is not interactivity-solidarity. Therefore every method of repair should create situations that facilitate discovering efforts and thus discovering our own contradicting intentions.

The demand to implement something unclear reminds me of the attempt to create a conditioned reflex in a dog so that it "will distinguish" between a circle and an ellipse. When the difference between the circle and an ellipse was very slight, the dog forgot everything he knew beforehand and then became restless. Apparently, the dog also needs a clear perception of what he is facing and he will prepare and respond accordingly (to salivate or not to salivate and so on).

From here we can perhaps understand why pathological states also cause cognitive atrophy and not only "emotional" disturbances. The dog forgot everything he knew. In the human being, as we have said, knowledge is incompatible with anxiety, with the state of internal contradiction, or in other words, the state in which one cannot find an effective response to external stimuli.

In acute states of disorder, the person wakes up tired in the morning, tired because while he is sleeping he also continues with his set behavior of contracted lumbar and occipital muscles. We have seen the vulnerability of these two areas and that every failed learning process will be expressed there. In these states there are sometimes cognitive difficulties. Good cognition sees the significant connection between the different elements. "Significant" in the sense of the relationship of the elements to each other and all their relationships to something whole. This is similar to the activity of the sensors and the effectors which increase their interactivity according to one conclusive goal, an intention that unites with action according to the situation.

I remember a fortyish year old man who came for help and reported that he listened to his voice from the side as though he were not the speaker.

The asymmetric principle had been destroyed in this individual (who functioned as a "normal" person in society). Obviously, the attempt to help could not simply focus on treating his vocal chords and his hearing.

Cognition and emotional value are interconnected in that every idea is accompanied by the emotional attitude of rejection or acceptance. The neurotic has a negative attitude in his self-use and consequently in his speech. He only feels "solidarity" with himself in the state of "noise" in which the contracted flexors do not allow for complete potent activity of the extensors. There are no clear processes of inhibition and coordination. The intention to do something potent arouses an action of defense and contraction of the flexors. The sympathetic system which is meant to prepare the organism for removal of the threat (the potent state is threatening because it is unfamiliar) is aroused but has nothing to do in the preparation created by this system and therefore there is no healing from the disturbance and no antagonistic action of the parasympathetic system. It seems to me that it would be worthwhile to check the connection between the state in which the antagonistic activity of these two systems is undermined, and different illnesses in the organism. In the sexual relations of the neurotic, consciousness intervenes at the moment of ejaculation (or orgasm for the woman). In ejaculation in healthy circumstances, the pelvis makes several reflexive movements so that the semen can penetrate deeply. The neurotic who is not used to following one organ (the asymmetric principle) feels threatened by totally "following" the pelvis. We have seen that in a vaguely threatening situation, consciousness "descends" to involvement with the details of performance and here too consciousness gets involved in the pelvis' reflex action and spoils it. This is similar to swallowing a bitter medicine while consciously involved in the details of swallowing, something that disturbs the swallowing reflex and makes swallowing the medicine impossible.

Some researchers claim that the neurotic cannot relate sexual functioning to the general scheme of self-image and that orgasm is threatening because it is as though there is a loss of self-image and clear boundaries. It seems to me that my explanation which is connected to destroying the asymmetric principle includes these claims as well. The adult who has not consolidated his own response to one organ (the asymmetric principle) has not really built clear boundaries since he has not learned to act with interactivity and solidarity for his own satisfaction. His body scheme is vague and blurry since childhood when there were two contradictory neuro-motor streams, that is to say, one of potency and one of defense. He is always in an elevated "state of preparation", sometimes remote and detached.

In my opinion, this is not about the inability of relating function to schema since in any case, there is no concern of losing the vagueness, but it is about the ignorance of moving according to the asymmetric principle in interactivity and solidarity to achieve sexual satisfaction that is primarily located in the sexual organ. The neurotic learns that this self-activation threatens his security.

When I sit near the piano and try to learn a section of J. S. Bach's *Partita*, what am I really doing? Am I clarifying and guiding myself through my fingers and ears or am I perhaps searching for value from others and in actuality negating myself? The answer to this question will become clear in the exploration of **grades of mind** of intention and action. The following example clarifies this concept: when I hear the voice of my crying baby I rush to help him, I do this as an impulsive action but the process actually has different stages.

First I hear the voice, then I discern a human voice (and not a cat voice, for example) then I discern the voice of an infant and then I discern that it is my son crying. In an anxious state, there is an impulsive neuro-motor response when the desire to implement something potent appears; the person is in a dulled state of mind with rather poor performance ability, over-involvement with details, with neuromotor contradictions in his behavior.

If I have a latent aspect of self-negation, this will be expressed in grades of mind of performance. For example, the pelvic movement that contradicts the movement of the bending of the knee towards the stomach while lying on the side. I want to move my knee but at the same time, I move the pelvis in a way that contradicts this "desire". Grades of mind can be discovered in the very moment of transition from intention to performance.

In this moment there is usually "parasitic preparation" that contradicts the movement that we want to realize and sometimes there is a moment of breath-holding as well. Has anyone checked how many times a day children hold their breath when they are trying to solve non-familiar math questions?

Chapter Five

Many people are confused about the concept of spontaneity and the concept of parasitic activity. When asked to do something, they do so immediately, which seems to be a spontaneous response, since it is immediate. Usually, an immediate response includes efforts connected with parasitic preparation that contrast with the requested aim. In this response there will be a sensation of poor involvement that will actually occur as a kind of reflex, an activity that happens in my body but is foreign to me, an activity that does not have total self-involvement.

We will see that spontaneity is the highest level in human behavior and has both the feeling of clarification in implementation and the feeling of total control between stimulation to inhibition grounded in rest and deep satisfaction. I remember the definition that one of my teachers gave to the terms "righteous" and "evil". The evil person surrendered to his heart alone while the righteous person holds his heart in his hands.

It seems to me that the definition of the righteous person is similar to the definition of the person who acts spontaneously. He is aware of his heartfelt feelings and facilitates them with the feeling that he controls the stimulation or inhibition of the inner process. In the sense of "Why so downcast, my soul, why disquieted within me?" (Psalms).

One can see unsuccessful education as a process that teaches the child to hide his potent intentions in mind-building and instead to "achieve" imaginary and ridiculous goals that bind him to the adult with chains of blurriness and helplessness. In comparing a neurotic-obsessive condition with a condition of pain, an interesting difference becomes apparent. In the experience of pain, I look into myself and experience the pain in a specific place in my body. The pain causes me to take an effective action, for example, I go to the doctor. I discern something in myself that causes me to organize an effective response. This is similar to the process of perception and sensation connected with external stimuli, a process of seeing within myself a possible response to the stimulus. In the process of fear there is also perception and sensation, that is to say, the inherent response to the external threat. This response enables me to decide whether to fight or to flee since it prepares the organism for vigorous action.

There is a sensation of wakefulness-choice because there is cause and effect – an action which may possibly cancel the threat or disturbance. This is not the case with anxiety; the feeling of danger stems from the person and is accompanied by a defensive response of contracting the flexors and a disturbance in the heart and diaphragm area. But this response that prepares the organism for vigorous action is unnecessary since there is no one to attack and no one to escape from. There is no effective action to take. The mind is not built for this state since its unity connects with **one meaning** that it gives the stimuli in a period of time that is connected with finding a possible response to the stimulus. In anxiety there is no unity of minds, no possible response and one cannot attribute one meaning to the stimuli whose source is unclear. Here again we can see why anxiety is incompatible with knowing. Knowing means distinguishing between the appropriate action and the mistaken action in relation to stimuli that affect the person, but in anxiety this discernment is impossible because one cannot see whether a specific action is appropriate or mistaken. There is no opportunity to take any action. The need for potent action is threatening since it is accompanied with a profound feeling of inability. Due to the threat, the defense mechanism is aroused and one cannot therefore not take potent measures or defensive action.

Chapter Five

Anxiety is, if so, the state of **no mind** and therefore it is not surprising that the anxious state can pass into a psychotic state, in which the person creates imaginary "meanings" and thus supposedly constructs his mind. All the different rituals are actions in which the person has a "meaningful response" to the "stimulus" that he creates. The need for unifying the mind is the most basic need and even people who suffer from schizophrenia have only one character at any given moment, a character with its own world and its own unique responses. From all this one can perhaps learn that anxiety is a dulled state (sometimes in anxiety, there is a feeling of drowsiness and detachment) and exists when there are two contradictory neuro-motor directions whose formation can be related to mistaken learning, the inherent desire for potency and a profound feeling of inability.

The factors reinforcing this inability are: effort, speed, dullness and the desire to stop when there is improvement. Performance is the revelation of the hidden psychic tendency. A person can say one thing and do something totally different. The fact that he says something consciously does not indicate what is going on inside. This will be revealed in action which always means movement.

The adult does not approve of most of the child's learning processes; he expects the child to do what he did and wants quick results without giving the child the means to achieve them. This leads to the formation of hidden messages since the child feels that their expression is dangerous. He limits and restricts his self-utilization and remains with a vague self-image detached from his own experiential world. Instead of awareness helping him look within and see clearly what is happening, it serves as a tool for creating "rational processes". This is sterile intellectualism that cannot generate anything except that which already is, that is to say, holding onto a broken crutch. In this context, it is difficult not to mention the child who hangs on to his mother and drags after her in "walking" which is a caricature of walking.

I remember when I was a substitute eighth grade teacher of arithmetic for several months in a school in Jerusalem. It was the best arithmetic class in the school. I asked one of the students to do a simple exercise - to divide the number 525 by the number 5. The student did the exercise easily and I think the whole class could have done so. Next, I asked the student to explain the operations that he used in division. He repeated the operations over and over and said 5 divided by 5 is 1 and he wrote the number 1 on the blackboard. I asked where did he take 5 from? We are talking about 500.

The student did not understand the question and, like the rest of the class, did not know how to answer. My attempts to clarify the meaning of the exercise met with the fierce opposition of the whole class.

Later both the parents and the supervisor showed their resistance to the strange teacher who undermined the successful image of their children. I was fired from my job when the supervisor realized that the children also had difficulties in other simple arithmetic exercises.

The quick demand for results may teach the child to connect learning with danger, effort and blows to his confidence. This child will need encouragement for every future challenge and will give up on something new **if he is not guaranteed success beforehand.** The separation between experience and consciousness reaches its peak in sick people who complain that something external is hurting them despite the fact that the pain is in and from their own body. They have lost the ability to connect between experience and consciousness; they do not recognize the pain as their own. Here one of the fundamental characteristics of the mind was destroyed; for example, I experience the fact of standing and I recognize that it is **I who am standing** which enables me to have control over what's happening even though I do not know how I do it. As for the sick person, even the pain does not facilitate organized action to insure his well-being and security. The same sick person has perhaps learned in early childhood that using his own interactivity and solidarity to satisfy his needs threatens his security.

It should be remembered that the young child is unaware of the process of being guided by the adult and cannot create his own alternatives. The way the infant teaches himself is inherent and includes the possibility of discovering something new, while protecting the interactivity and solidarity, or in other words, in the process of walking into the unknown he is able to regulate his own well-being.

As we have seen the conclusive intention is dull, consciousness gets involved in the details of performance, that is to say, there is a need to be involved in the question of how.

We will mention in passing that this is one of the difficulties in remedial teaching. On one hand, one doesn't want the person involved in the how, in the details of performance, and on the other hand, we must be involved in the question of how, because this facilitates discovery and the clarification of contradictory intention. (I will discuss this question in the chapter on Cure.)

The involvement in the details of performance is characteristic of the neurotic, he is involved in the act of breathing when he speaks, he is involved in the muscles of his hands and fingers when he writes and so on. The same abstract quality in musical playing or singing or creative thought is the state in which there is no involvement in the details of the performance. Attention wanders in a simple flow and there is a clear feeling of my own clear presence. When I play (a musical instrument), my intention is not to hit the keyboards or to sit on the chair, or to look at the notes and put my fingers on the right place on the keyboard. My intention is none of these actions and even doing them together is not my intention but nonetheless they serve my intention that is to express something, understand something. Therefore, in order to reach an abstract level, one must establish the details of performance during the learning process in wakefulness choice which then sink into the unconscious, creating the possibility of a higher purpose. If the actions were acquired in a learning process which had an inner contradiction in the neuromotor system, they would not quietly sink into the unconscious because an open question remains - lack of confidence and worry over the actual performance cannot generate higher level intentions. A deep feeling of inability does not go hand in hand with aspirations.

The neurotic state shows that the person did not learn to use himself asymmetrically; while safeguarding interactivity and solidarity, he did not develop the ability of organized and variegated action in the time-space dimension and consequently the whole process of abstraction connected with psychic integration and intention is not well-functioning. Abstraction is impossible without psychic integration and intention and these become blurred when the ability for "primary action" is destroyed.

It seems to me that one of the great achievements of the organism is its ability to utilize solutions from the past in the present and future. This is where the question of compulsive activity arises connected to learning which has limited the use of self, creating only one possible impulsive and undifferentiated response to something new. When the experience of the past is acquired in an emotional pressure cooker, the ability to know which part of past experience is appropriate or inappropriate to the present will not develop. The child's use of self shrinks because he has learned that his body behavior endangers the love that he can and wants to receive. A person does not distinguish what he does not "want" to distinguish and he does not "want" to distinguish when he does not have a likely response to the external stimulus. Anxiety is not in accord with knowing because it does not facilitate the state of "primary action"; the non-successful past experience stands in contrast to the potent learning inherent in us since evolution. The neurotic's feeling of compulsion is connected with his not having a "primary purpose", doing one thing on a different cognitive level that has an element of intention and all other factors respond appropriately to the action.

This is the state of comprehension which was defined as the possibility of seeing how the parts relate to the whole or, in other words, how the parts contribute to the fact that the whole is one whole. This state of comprehension is identical, in my opinion, to the feeling of free will. The anxious state has a vague and hardened element, purposeless and senseless, and lacks the possibility of choosing between arousal and inhibition.

The same outburst of different senses that reinforce each other towards the conclusive result, that exists in developed animals, provides the possibility for change according to changing circumstances in the process and the possibility of seeing if it actually achieves the cumulative result. This is the beginning of the possibility of knowledge, cause and effect, understanding the relationship between the parts and the whole. Failed learning jumbled this basic characteristic in that it did not facilitate one intention in a time period and thus destroyed the foundation of "primary action".

We have seen that the individual cannot be the site for two meanings simultaneously and meanings is defined as intentions in the sense of possible response. In failed learning, the intention of implementing something potent (this comes from the force of evolution) immediately arouses the neuro-motor process of defense. The nervous system receives contradictory messages and the person is in a blurry and threatened state. In this state there can be no clear knowing with a deep echo in which the whole organism participates.

One can describe psychotic states as an extreme result of deligitmization of learning and the child's self-use, so much so that the child's "security" requires him to determine that **it is not he who is doing this.** In these states, the person seems to have disappeared, he is not present. The same basic principle of existence of mind connected to control over the action and awareness of the action is no longer viable.

Learning is a process in which the higher hierarchies refine and perfect the response, but the successful process must occur without harming the child's interactivity and solidarity and without limiting his whole presence in the action. We do not claim that a thermometer knows that it is now cold, since the cold does not awaken in the thermometer the feeling that moves it to do something (wear a coat); consequently, a person only knows something if it arouses within him a specific feeling.

CHAPTER SIX
Vocal Expression and its Centrality in Knowing and Experiencing

From the moment that the infant uses his voice for gratification, he is actually using it as a language, that is to say, as a means of creating a connection with the other. In these early stages the infant does not perceive himself as an entity separate from his mother and from the environment, but nevertheless he activates himself in interactivity and solidarity. All the systems connected with vocal expression function in complete harmony and in accordance with the infant's intention, whether it be expression of pain, anger, laughter, demand for attention and so on. The pressure in the diaphragm corresponds with the pressure in the larynx, the vocal chords are fully coordinated with these two organs, and the various cavities and different organs amplify the voice accordingly. The infant does not plan how much air to inhale or exactly when to begin to inhale and exhale air so as to produce a sound. He also does not plan his jaw and tongue movements. In these early stages, there is rarely hoarseness or fatigue, the infant can continue to cry for a long time and his voice will remain clear and rich. There is rich movement of the torso and coordination between the chest movement and the diaphragm and stomach, all the organs respond in accord with the infant's aim of using his voice to gratify himself. He learns, for example, that by making an intense sound he gets food and assuages the disturbing feeling of hunger.

The connection between organic feelings and what is expressed in the infant's voice is clear. The pain he feels is expressed in different aspects of his voice such as: intensity, melody, range, declamation, and so on.

They inform the mother of what he wants and whether he is satisfied or unsatisfied. This complex performance of producing a sound and using it organically is an inborn ability and there is no one who can teach the infant to make this sound.

In order to teach this, one would have to calculate precisely which muscles to contract and at what times, what air pressure is necessary at every moment and how much air has to be inhaled for every one of the different vocal expressions and above all to **teach the connection between the specific organic sensation and this or another vocal expression.**

Clearly this is impossible and nonetheless the infant has the ability to do this in complete harmony serving his intention of achieving gratification. This is a basic trait inherent in every living organism namely the coordinated movement which serves the need for continued existence.

In slightly later stages, the infant does not necessarily use his voice to demand food or bathing but as a means of self-gratification, in the actual use of the vocal chords. Producing sounds is connected with eating and therefore is a pleasant association. There are those who claim that this is one of the infant's ways of auto-erotic gratification. The repetition makes the activity easier to do and the infant draws pleasure from this as well.

A characteristic of the infant's use of his voice is the rich movement in the torso of all the mechanisms that contribute to voice production and the correct well-coordinated work division and pattern of short inhalations and relatively long productions.

From the vantage point of the natural sciences, the mechanisms connected with voice production have been used correctly; however, the infant does not intend to use the mechanism properly, he just intends to gratify himself by using his voice.

We will generalize and comment that just when the use of the body in the gravitational field is what is required according to consistent physical logic, exactly then there is a chance for the fullest clearest expression and the sense of freedom of choice. I will discuss this matter later. It seems to me, that the act of breathing is dictated by the reflexes connected to the amount of carbon dioxide in the blood. The diaphragm muscles are part of the autonomic system that is not usually connected with a voluntary-conscious act. The diaphragm is sensitive to every situation, be it a threat or a feeling of satisfaction and functions accordingly. We have seen that in threatening situations, there is a disturbance in the area of the diaphragm and consequently there is breath-holding or a disturbance in the breathing rhythm. There is much movement of the diaphragm in states of joy or sadness, and little movement in states of embarrassment or worry. In fearful states, the coordination between the stomach movement and the chest movement is affected, and the production duration is short; in states of anger, the production duration is long. In later stages of life, even remembering different emotional situations can produce the appropriate response in the diaphragm and the other parts of the body that can expand will respond appropriately, an example being nasal resonance. In pathological states, when the difference between current and past reality is blurred, there may be an appropriate diaphragmatic response to past events because something in the current situation jostles a memory from the past. This reinforces the whole situation of the past. Sometimes in a pathological state, one cannot deconstruct the past into its elements and see which part fits the current situation.

Chapter Six

One definition of a mentally healthy person is someone who is aware of what is happening around him and responds to these demands without violating his integrity. Speech and voice are the tools and also the result of the process of adjustment. The infant connects with reality with these tools and tries to adjust; at an older age he uses these tools according to how he adjusted to his environment. As described earlier, in the initial stage the infant does not violate his integrity, he functions in an interactive and solidarity way, but is still unaware of what is happening around him. He does not yet perceive himself as separate from his mother and cannot respond to her demands as such. The objects look very blurry and he does not yet have a crystallized world of concepts.

Speech, which is a tool for communication, will reveal the frustration and indirectness of unsuccessful adaptation. An effective sound is a sound that relates to the intention of the speaker. The speaker lets the listener know what he (the speaker) thinks, how he feels and how he feels in relation to what he thinks.

In the adjustment phase, the infant may hold his breath and make spastic movements of raising his larynx as a way of expressing frustration. If the adult's response to this behavior is positive, the infant may develop this as a permanent response.

It seems to me that the main process in development is the infant's gradual perception of himself as separate and distinct from his mother and from the environment. We have seen that this process is primarily implemented through the collaboration of the skeletal muscles and the teleceptors with which the infant acquires control over moving his body in the gravitational field. Together with this, he gains control over the objects around him, and thus creates within himself the conceptual world and an awareness that the objects in his environment, including his mother, are not inside him but on the outside.

This process seems quite difficult and in its course, the child's interactivity and solidarity may get scrambled.

Neurologically, one can describe the child's learning process as a process in which the high hierarchies at first cause inhibition of certain reflexes that are only restarted at a later stage. This matter is connected with the myelinization of the dendrites and the axons in the brain that is first implemented in the low hierarchies and only afterwards in the high ones. We have seen that the function of the high hierarchies is to refine and improve the response to the environment; perhaps "to refine and improve" means to respond more precisely, and more gradually with the possibility of more order in the time-space dimension and the goal of more clarification. And here the critically important question - will this be a process of refinement and improvement or perhaps a process in which the use of those reflexes that connect between the organic sensations and the vocal mechanisms is brutally stopped? Does one, by being overprotective, develop a distorted use of the mechanism as in the example above - in which the child holds his breath and makes spastic movements of the larynx. There is a rather slight and fine line between those stimuli that help the child refine and improve his response and those stimuli that may detach him, God forbid, from his ability to authentically express himself, or from the ability to use himself with interactivity and solidarity as an individuated organism capable of negotiating with his environment. The ability to negotiate with the environment from a position of potency is connected to efficient moving of the body in the gravitational field and consequently creating the conceptual world and the feeling of "behavioral time". Interestingly, refinement and improvement are expressed in intentions that are articulated in peripheral organs, such as: writing and playing music with the fingers, speech with movements of the oral cavity and the tongue and so on.

The ability to pronounce vowels and consonants develops gradually from relatively simple consonants, producing "be" (as in "better") and "de" (as in "delicious") to the more complex consonants such as "k" (as in "king") or "ge" (as in "get"). The first of the vowels is "a" (as in "alpha", which according to our sages is pronounced in the lungs) until the more complex vowels such as "o" and "ee". The formation of more complex vowels and consonants means a more complex system of inhibitions, that is to say creating an element of more complex order in the time-space dimension. One has to be careful that this creation of order does not remove the reflexive connection between vocal expression and organic feeling and that the vocal mechanism is not used harmfully to achieve "virtual security" by upsetting the child's interactivity and solidarity. Overly rigid learning under heavy emotional pressure will create inhibitions that leave no space for dynamism and flexibility and disrupt the reflex functions that connect the organic feelings and motor articulation and thus limit the experiencing and expression. This learning will indeed lead to knowledge but knowledge with only one option, knowledge that conjures up the feeling of holding tight onto one way of doing things, which is defined above as a state of anxiety.

The "information", if so, will be accompanied by anxiety which is incompatible with true knowledge since it does not allow for change in implementation and inventiveness.

The fact that the child learns to clarify, refine and perfect his intentions must not be at the expense of the reflexes that connect him with organic experience.

We have seen that this process of inhibition and order is unconscious and every effort at conscious dictation will only cause a disturbance of the proper functioning of things. As we have already seen, telling a person to use his tongue in a specific way creates a neurotic state in which consciousness "descends" into the details of performance. If the tongue isn't coordinated, something is lacking in the speaker's intention and perception of self. The non-coordinated tongue movement is not a cause but rather a result and when the perpetuating cause disappears, it will disappear.

Similarly, the diaphragm functions according to the speaker's reflexes and intentions. Every attempt to teach improved functioning of the diaphragm by exercising the diaphragm is basically mistaken. One should facilitate a return to the state in which the reflexive connection between diaphragm functioning and the different emotional states is created anew. One can help clarify the speaker's intentions by clarifying and enriching his self-image and by getting rid of rigid, a priori positions expressed in muscular movements that do not allow for reflex activity. One cannot activate a reflex via consciousness, just the opposite - involvement of consciousness just disturbs the reflex action (see the discussions on swallowing a pill and ejaculation).

If a sound is produced with the weak and inappropriate "support" of the diaphragm, it is erroneous to tell the student "to get support" using the diaphragm. The muscles that activate the diaphragm are part of the autonomous system and demanding their activation is actually an unclear demand that only undermines their coordinated functioning and limits the range of response.

The student will learn that only with uncertain efforts in the upper abdominal area can he produce a sound. Instead of being absorbed in the developing stream of thoughtful and emotional expression, he will be rigidly involved with the details of performance, clutching at a straw, which can only lead to further clutching at a straw.

Now let us try to examine why the diaphragm sometimes does not function reflexively and coordinated with the speaker's intention.

A characteristic of the mind is its ability to utilize the organs of the body so that the person's intention does not contradict reflexes. The fixation reflex of the eye which (in a healthy person) results in the eye tracking after a moving object does not contradict the person's ability to turn his gaze on demand, that is to say, voluntarily. In some pathological cases a person cannot turn his gaze on demand and nonetheless the eye follows "on its own" after the moving object according to the "fixation reflex". The fixation reflex is adjacent to the "roof of the brain" far from the area of "voluntary control" of vision. A successful learning process allows for voluntary control of turning the gaze without harming the reflex action. For example, the hunter's eye tracking the bird in the sky is not disturbed as he maneuvers his rifle to mark the moving goal just as our eyelids' reflexive blinking does not disturb our reading. The question arises - why doesn't the eye's fixation reflex disrupt the process of the infant's adaptation to his environment and why do the reflexes connected with the diaphragmatic activity and vocal expression often collapse?

As we have seen, the reflexes that activate the diaphragm bind its functioning to different emotional states. If, for example, an adult asks the child to control his emotions than the child learns to restrict the rich movement of the diaphragm connected with the range of emotional responses. If expression of all the feelings that surface when something new is presented is not legitimated, then the very latent ties between the child's emotional world and his diaphragmatic activity will be destroyed, sometimes irrevocably with no chance of rehabilitation, and the "learned" thing will be perceived as detached from and in contradiction to his inner feelings.

In correct learning which fully validates all feelings, the child gradually and unconsciously learns a more refined and better use of the diaphragm for a more discriminating vocal and verbal expression of surfacing processes and thoughts. This resembles the hunter whose maneuvering of the rifle in his hand does not disturb the eye's fixation reflex as it continues to track the bird moving in the sky. In successful learning, the child learns to coordinate between the diaphragm functioning and the activities of the other speech organs so as to articulate his thoughts without being detached from the feelings accompanying the learning process that is essentially a moving towards the unknown. Delegitimization of the experiencing that is connected to this moving towards the unknown which is expressed in the demand for too-early results destroys the very reflexes that connect between the emotional world and the movement of the diaphragm and therefore diaphragmatic functioning becomes very restricted and emotions are inhibited and denied. The word that is meant to crystallize the latent process of clarification of this experiencing becomes an empty vessel, a dry tree, a strange thing. Not for naught is reading comprehension one of the most painful problems in our educational system. Why would a sane person want to "understand" something that destroys the very emotional and motor associations that are his essence as a living creature?

It is apparently not coincidental that the ancient Greeks called the diaphragm the same name as the human brain (fren). In Hebrew, too, the word "*sarafim-machshavot*" (immersed in thought) has the same root as the word *sarephet* (diaphragm).

We must remember that if the neuromotor basis slips, then the adjacent psychic reality cannot exist. Therefore, restricting diaphragmatic activity can cause a narrowing of the person's psychic reality at an older age.

However, since the child must speak and respond to the teacher's questions, he does so with the little air under the clavicle that barely suffices to create a vibration in the vocal chords. This sensation causes the throat, jaw, lips and tongue to make a contrived (purposeless) effort to compensate for the lack of air stemming from the poor diaphragmatic activity. The child's pleasing, clear and rich voice sound disappears almost entirely when he goes to school. The same wonderful coordination that connects the varied emotional reality with the interactive activity of the diaphragm and all the participating factors in voice production and speech is sometimes harmed irreparably while at the same time the ability to connect the experiential world and the structured concept is also affected. As a result, the processes intended to bring us to a better understanding of our reality are disrupted.

We have defined effort as the state in which more than necessary work is invested to implement an action. In activity of the diaphragm that becomes more restricted than necessary, too much force is invested in the speech organs and the right division of labor is destroyed. Instead of most of the energy for speech coming from rich breathing activity, unnecessary energy is invested in the more delicate organs that are just meant to refine and improve expression (create resonance, speech movements, vowels and consonants). These organs cannot compensate for the inadequate energy that is a result of faulty breathing and consequently these fine mechanisms are destroyed. Ulcers develop on the vocal chords which are overexerted due to the inadequate breathing. A similar scenario – instead of doing a job with the strength in my hands and my body, I am told to only use my fingers. This will obviously damage the fingers' connective tissue.

The unnecessary overexertion of the delicate organs lowers their level of differentiation and consequently, there are times when no sound can be produced.

The strain of the incorrect distribution of labor results in a disruption of expression and a blurred self-image. An interesting circularity occurs. The teacher demanded the separation of the learning process from the experiential world, which resulted in the restriction of the diaphragmatic activity and consequently, an incorrect distribution of labor, overexertion and blurred ability of expression and thus a blurring of self-image. The teacher's demand which essentially restricts the inner world, generates blurry expression and an undifferentiated self-image. The child will learn to connect expression and thinking with a mistaken division of labor and with effort which maintains the condition of blurred knowledge and experience. The child will learn that the learning process and intellectual concepts are contrary to his well-being, to the state in which a connection exists between his psychic reality and the motor expression of the diaphragm's movement.

Chapter Six

Anatomically, the breathing muscles are connected with the hips and with the neck. The muscles of the diaphragm are connected to the lumbar vertebrae and the muscles of the chest are connected to the occipital vertebrae. We have seen that the lumbar and occipital vertebrae are susceptible to injury in the adaptation process to the gravitational field. In unsuccessful adaptation the division of labor between the skeletal muscles will be incorrect and the occipital and lumbar area will be overexerted. In some cases, the head will sink onto the thorax, rendering free movement impossible. The occipital muscles will greatly exert themselves to turn the gaze forward. The effort in the lumbar area will render full and rich movement of the diaphragm impossible. The effort in the occipital area will cause a decrease of discernment in the area and it will be impossible to discern the exertions of the tongue, larynx, jaw etc. The education to conceal the experience that causes non-successful adaptation to the gravitational field will cause, if so, a quite pathetic vocal and breathing expression. Attempts at emotional expression at an older age will contradict the person's habitual expression and instead of authentic expression there will be exertion and closures. The parasitic forces that operate in the jaw, tongue and larynx will prevent the free flow of the voice outward. There will be a sensation of "lack of air" which is actually the lack of coordination of the activity of the diaphragm and the activity of the speech organs, which will cause the air to be trapped in the respiratory system. There will be a raised larynx and jaw movement and a parasitic action in the tongue muscles that will seemingly give "support" to the sound but which is no more than a cessation of the free flow of air. The performer will imagine that he is producing a big sound that is actually a small and tense sound. The exertion from this inaccurate distribution of labor perpetuates this inability; this type of person identifies with what he has learned - performance and expression are achieved with effort. Therefore it is odd to think that repair can come from learning to use the diaphragm, tongue, jaw and larynx correctly for we are discussing disrupted coordination of all these organs which blurs intention and self-image because of pathetic breathing and unsuccessful adjustment to the gravitational field.

In actuality, blurring of intention, non-successful adjustment to the gravitational field and restriction of the activity of the diaphragm and thorax area are different aspects of the same thing and a result of too-early demand which caused a detachment of consciousness from the interactive solidarity processes, that facilitates the right division of labor and a simple connection between the emotional and the motor reality, that facilitates a clear feeling of self image and the enrichment and discernment of the use of self.

An effective voice relates to the speaker's intention that lets the listener know what he thinks and feels. An effective voice requires, if so, that there be clear intention and clear self-perception linked with the ability to discern what I feel or what my relationship is to the idea I express with my voice.

Singing may serve as a voluntary recollection, an echo of the pure satisfaction of primary vocalization. This auto-erotic activity liberates the accumulated repressed tensions. We sing to express or create pleasing sounds and not primarily to arouse admiration. Is our educational system like this? Do we learn to express in good faith, to create pleasing sounds? Or perhaps we want to be valued by others through our singing, to earn our profoundly lacking sense of worth since we have a profound feeling of lack of capability.

Chapter Six

The trend of searching for value will be expressed in grades of mind. In voice production, a feeling of effort will be connected with contradictory trends; on one hand, the desire to "express" and on the other hand, a deep feeling of the inability to express. There will be muscular activity that contradicts the effort to express and create a rich sound, which as soon as it is conscious, we will perhaps be able to get rid of and thus start the process of clarification and more authentic and rich expression. Interesting to note in this context that there is much more muscular activity in deep breathing than in shallow breathing, but in shallow breathing there is a feeling of effort due to the contrasting directions of the different muscles.

Usually one can discern three major factors in poor use of the voice: inappropriate use of power, incorrect pitch, ineffective breathing. These three factors are actually three aspects of the same thing. In poor posture, with its primary effort in the lumbar and occipital area, effective breathing is impossible. The division of labor in voice production (between the massive muscles and the more refined muscles) will be incorrect and consequently inappropriate force will be used. It will also be impossible to find the right pitch since the torso cannot support the sound and the parasitic activity of the jaw, tongue and larynx covers over this inability.

The appropriate pitch will be found with a correct division of labor and this requires perfect posture and clear intention. It should be remembered that purely mechanically, producing a melodic sound is a process in which a strong current of air is directed to the vocal chords and without perfect posture the torso cannot contain the opposing pressure inside. The sunken chest area cannot contain the air and produce the flexible breathing pulse necessary for producing the movements of speech. Speech vowels that are not crystallized are one of the signs of parasitic forces in the speech organs and the trend towards concealment. Perfect artistic expression is simple and direct without the twisting paths characteristic of non-successful adjustment process. Imperfect posture is the reason for parasitic efforts in the speech organs and for the state of a non-closing of the vocal cords, that is to say, only partial use of the voice muscles which causes fatigue, ulcers and hoarseness. In the unsuccessful adjustment process, the person omits several emotional-motor positions from his repertoire and thus limits and impoverishes himself further.

The movement repertoire shrinks, the interactivity is disrupted and consequently the expressive ability becomes poorer. The trend of concealment, connected with the unsuccessful adaptation is expressed in the raised larynx and the straining jaw, that work against the parasitic efforts in the diaphragm in the effort to express something I deeply feel and believe that I cannot express and the sunken chest area only contributes another layer in the lack of coordination. The body does not inhale independently after the voice production and inhalation becomes conscious. There is a feeling of something shut, lack of air and inability to support the sound, something that drags additional effort in its wake that cause even weaker ability and on and on. This is not a state of increasing clarity but a state of involvement with actions and conscious dictation on how to act.

The grades of mind that appear in the form of these efforts reveal the performer's true relationship to the performed material and to himself and can teach something of his true intention that is usually connected with the search for value and sympathy accompanied by a deep feeling of inability.

Chapter Six

There are three components to vocal expression:
a. Presentation – what one wants to say
b. Expression – reveals something of the speaker
c. Appeal – aims to arouse a response in the listener (the addressee)

In pathological states the component of expression is very confused and the third component non-existent. Speech has a monotonous quality and the listener does not seem to be addressed by the voice.

Let us stop momentarily and think if our educational system encourages or perhaps blocks the development of these components. Is the child encouraged to reveal his feelings when he presents a solution to the question? Do we educate to arouse a response in the listener (aside from the response of receiving his immediate approval)? Are we educated to be listening addresses to the other?

I remember a case brought to my attention of a six-year-old child who was hoarse and severely strained his voice. The appropriate medical treatments did not help. The father of this child was a salesman accustomed to talking in order to try and convince others to purchase his merchandise but he himself was not prepared to listen to other people speaking. This child had no address for his own speech and so he used pressure and effort in the hope that he would be listened to, which caused a malfunctioning of the vocal mechanism. We have seen that the breathing and voice production of the infant are totally coordinated and that this coordination may well be adversely affected when the child is concerned about revealing something about himself as well as when there is no listening address. The sentences will usually end with almost no remaining air and the child will try to compensate with his delicate speech organs. In a successful learning process, the voice gradually serves the speech and content until it becomes emotional background. In pathological states, voice production is conscious and does not seem to be in accord with the speaker's content. This conscious involvement sometimes causes a conscious involvement with breathing as well as the unsuccessful effort of planning the amount of air necessary for the sentence. Singers with inadequate or incorrect voice training become involved in producing a large sound instead of focusing on expression and clarification, using their voice as emotional background.

When the purpose of communication is vague, the coordination between breathing and production suffers. Clarifying intention that is connected with the process of clarifying self-image and enriching use of self will help in the coordinated activation of the whole mechanism. Breathing will begin automatically when the person plans to speak and the appropriate amount of air is inhaled.

I would like to stop the discussion of the topics presented in this chapter until now and address a seemingly separate topic - **the use of words to create sentences.**

The accepted opinion is that a person thinks using words, that is to say, the thinking process is verbal. Is this really true? A person expresses his thoughts using words that he chooses; he then builds sentences from these words. The sentence has a structure and a melody appropriate to the expressed thought. This occurs without the person consciously planning the structure, the appropriateness of the melody and without rehearsals prior to speaking. When a person speaks freely he does not even know beforehand what word he will use next in the sentence and nonetheless the right word usually appears, fitting the sentence structure and the accompanying melody.

Chapter Six

In my opinion, from the moment a person "chose" certain words, the **thinking process actually ended.** The process is intended to suit the word to the content that the person wants to express, but is this content also a word? If so how is the word chosen? Ultimately there is a need to fit certain words to the content that cannot be a word, that is to say, one adjusts between a word and an entity that is not a word. If so, what is this entity if it isn't a word?

We are meant to choose the appropriate word and so let us examine for a moment the selection process. When I want to choose a shirt, for example, how do I do so? Usually I choose a shirt in terms of size, shape, color and so on, that is to say, I choose a shirt with things that are not actually shirt. This is the case with a word, we are meant to choose a word with the help of concepts that are not words. If so the process of verbal expression is not conscious; is it at all rational? In a rational process we draw conclusions from assumptions using valid and fair rules. But this process occurs in sentences that are composed of words that we do not know how we chose. We do not have the interior experience of the process of choice just as we do not have the interior experience of all the expansive neuro-motor activity connected with moving our body in the gravitational field. All that I know is that it is I who am talking, that it is I who am hunting in order to get something. If so, the goal must be known from the start since one cannot otherwise explain why we take a step in this direction and not in another direction, why this word was chosen and not another and how the appropriate sentence structure and appropriate melody were created.

Russell was apparently right when he claimed that to be meaningful means to intend. If the goal is known beforehand, so then what is renewed in the verbal claim? Are we only involved in tautologies? Are we coming to a "new" planet and finding footprints that later turn out to be our footprints? Don't we determine the verdict first and only afterwards use the appropriate sections to justify and "explain" it?

Evolution created new things that did not exist before, in a process that, as we have seen, can be explained only a posteriori. There would be no point in creating the possibility of mind in man, which is apparently one of the peaks of evolution, if there were no existential advantage, that is, the possibility of absorbing hints and the slightest of hints from our surrounding reality and understanding how these hints relate to one another and how they all create and relate to one homogeneous reality, with which we can align ourselves so as to insure our safety and survival.

If so, let us return for a moment to the issue of learning to use the body in the gravitational field. In these early stages, the infant creates his mind, in the sense of building his unity from his own many parts, the ability to independently differentiate his distinctness from the environment, the ability to absorb signs from the environment and to create the possibility of uniting himself facing the environment. Building a rich and unified mind is possible but not necessary since we have seen that in a non-successful learning process the skills connected with moving the body in the gravitational field, the traits that are the essence of the mind are likely to become jumbled. Successful adaptation to the gravitational field will result in a higher level of differentiation of kinesthetic signs, and a clearer perception of self; it will lead to a clearer perception of the environment, and allow the person an interior experience of how his own different parts create and relate to himself as a whole, how the coordinated action of the different organs will bring the hoped-for result and simultaneously assist in its clarification. He will experience the simple connection of

Chapter Six

means and goals, or in other words, causes and effects. He will find a state of dynamic balance without eliminating the possibility of any actions or feelings a priori. It should be remembered that the word is a new phenomena in evolutionary concepts and was created only after man successfully adapted to the gravitational field, giving him an existential advantage.

In saying a verbal sentence, as in moving towards the goal of gratification, **something has to be clarified during the implementation** so that there is a possibility of change in the process of doing from the perspective of looking outward and listening inward.

CHAPTER SEVEN
Art as Cure

Bergson believes that there is a struggle for unity within the body and that the brain assumes an indispensable role in this struggle.

I would add to this - not only the brain, but also the mind plays an essential part in the struggle for unity - not only in the body but in the human being's whole psychic-physical entity.

I think that in science, as in art, this struggle for unity is fully expressed, since the human being uses them in the search for **a model of his mind in the world**, a model that allows for his existence as one whole entity (see chapter on Psychic Integration and the Concept of Mind). In science, the subject of deconstructing the inanimate whole in nature into its parts and finding the connections between the parts and themselves, and between the parts and the whole, is central. The unity of the whole as such stems from our discovery of these connections. In the study of the mind, especially the state of the finite mind, it becomes possible to see these relationships between the whole and its parts. Many components are within reach of one intention and the perception exists that **I am the one** who realizes the intention and that this I has the experience of control over the action, which is the realization of the intention. The I is one, since there are many different faculties which reinforce each other towards realization of the final cause.

The principle of the unity of the human self stems from the fact that in the human being there are different faculties including the teleceptors, the muscles, and the internal organs that function interactively. As we have

Chapter Seven

seen in earlier chapters, in one time period a person has the opportunity of doing only one "primary thing", which is done on a different level of cognition and contains an element of intention. Arguably, the concern of science and art is in principle identical - a process of examining and clarifying and learning to recognize different parts of the whole with the goal of revealing it as such and achieving a better understanding of it and its latent possibilities. Both help us momentarily get rid of those very parasitic forces that attach themselves to our core and shape "our personality". These forces were acquired in experience that always contained an undermining of the legitimacy of the learning process and a shaking up of our foundation as psycho-physical beings who function in an interactive- solidarity manner.

According to Sartre, a good play is a play in which, when something is happening on stage, something is revealed about the characters who become more familiar and clearer to us. When we leave a good play we feel that we "know" the characters. Art, then, is the refinement, essence and formulation of situations in which there is a more profound and daring attempt to reveal the totality, than in daily life, which consequently creates a clearer feeling of wakefulness choice and self-clarification. The theatre presents the audience with a slice of life that, on one hand, is very familiar while, on the other hand, has elements of vitality and clarification and presence that are usually not part of daily life. Art answers a profound need since, as we have already analyzed, it enables the existence of the mind in its full meaning and sets us face to face with ourselves in a clearer and more resolved fashion. From the perspective of the artist – and the observer - the need for art may actually be the need to be within the process of deconstructing the whole into its parts and constructing it again, in the attempt to let the whole be revealed as whole every time anew. This process provides the feeling of recovery since good art allows for more clarity and self-selection and the experience of wakefulness choice. Thus, the most important principle in art is the principle of unity within multiplicity, creating unity as a dynamic process and not something static or a priori, just as the essence of the mind is unity within multiplicity. **The mind, like a work of art, is on the one hand, so present, its presence so clear and definite, and on the other hand, so elusive.**

Sartre describes this beautifully when he says that when he listens to music blaring from a record player, its presence is so clear and influence so powerful and yet, it is not contained within any of the objects in the room he is in. Even if he breaks the record player and the record, says Sartre, he will not be able to find or touch the music itself. A creation of art, according to Sartre, is lacking actuality and the actor who embodies the character also becomes unreal in this role. He is totally absorbed in the illusion and derives his inspiration from the unreal. He uses his real body and limbs to act out intention that comes from the illusory and the unreal. So too, the mind will not be discovered in any research conducted by someone in the natural sciences on the human brain and body because the researcher will only discover objects whose connection with the mind is at the center of the psycho-physical problem that has occupied humankind for over two thousand years.

We have seen in earlier chapters that the developed animal advances towards its goal (food, sexual union, etc.) with all its faculties geared towards mutual reinforcement and then the animal adapts its movements according to the changing conditions. Man's psycho-physical unity has, as we have already seen, survival value, and in art, **man transforms this unity into the actual central matter and thus evolves further.**

Chapter Seven

Art also has goals but these are imaginary goals that are elucidated in the process of performance. In a play the question of the hero's real desires can arise; does he really act towards achieving his goal and intention? Tragic or dramatic situations in the theatre can be linked to this question of the hero's intention: Is it clear to him? Is he in the sway of forces that are not really his true will? The central question in the natural sciences is **what is the situation now?** In the human sciences and in art, the question is **what do I want now,** what is my intention now?

The process experienced by the character in the play is transmitted inspirationally to the viewers who also undergo a similar process of searching, clarification and refinement. The character's unclear state and unclear intention, is actually an interpretation of the state of the viewer, as well as some process of self-examination.

Recovery is actually a condition of returning to the mind in the discerning sense of the word, as defined in earlier chapters.

Art is abstraction of the process in which the animal realizes intention and satisfaction (food, coupling) and in art, **the very process of creating the situation of finite mind is the satisfaction**, the feeling of creating a clearer I, whose intention becomes clearer through attempts to realize something, is the goal.

Therefore in art one can discuss imaginary time that is created in this process of setting abstract goals and attempting to realize them. (This can be seen clearly in music, theatre and dance, in the states of creating the need for a solution or in states of tension and relaxation.)

In inanimate nature, one cannot find any intention. Intention is something connected with the animate and with man. Alfred Einstein summarizes his book on Mozart - Mozart's music creates a feeling that the universe doesn't have a mass, so too intention doesn't have a mass. In this sense, art is also an experience of a quasi-triumph over the obstacles of instrumental objects in the world and consequently there is a refining of the intention and a refining of man's communication with self and with the other.

If art and science are meant to provide a model of the human condition, then they must fulfill the basics of human existence. For example, as we have already seen, in speech, like in walking toward a destination, I do not experience the process of choosing a word or choosing the next step but nevertheless I have within me the clear experience that it is I who am hunting or speaking and I have control over my words or my steps and my path; I am in a direction that becomes clear to me as I try to realize it and I have within me the experience that I want to continue speaking or walking. Four basic components of regular human activity are expressed in art and in scientific performance at their best:
1. Experiencing of the self as fully involved in doing and acting.
2. Feeling of control over my actions
3. Being in the tendency that is clarified as it is realized
4. Feeling of the need and desire to continue in the action, despite the obstacles along the way.

We must ask ourselves how to train the young artist and researcher so that they have these qualities. Clearly involvement in activities and training of actions that can only be done one way or in a way that only emphasizes specific activity in a specific organ is basically erroneous. It cannot be about moving this or that limb in a manner dictated by external, mechanical and foreign forces. The connection between art and the healing process becomes apparent here, **relocating the person in himself as a whole.**

A person's feeling of dissociation and estrangement from his body are pathological signs. The inability to act as a complete whole in the process of clarification is characteristic of every situation needing repair. The art of performance at its best, in its being so demanding in the sense of total use of the self, can thus be a healing tool. This unity between the psychic and physical space is the embodiment of recovery in the sense of **one unity that functions in the world to achieve its satisfaction.** The material that the student has absorbed must be allowed to calmly sink into the realm of the unconscious, so as to facilitate higher aspirations. In interactivity-solidarity, intention reaches the height of clarity, there is no excess and more and more aspirations are generated.

When we watch a great artist at work, we feel purity in that there is nothing superfluous or in that everything is part of the clarification process. The healing process in art stems from the refinement and crystallization of intentions as opposed to the blurring of intention and self-image in daily life. The basis of the mind is one meaning in one period of time; art makes this possible and brings the person back to being one whole united by time, helped by the unity of the experience of the moment. In this special situation in human existence, intention and action become one with no screen between them.

Beethoven's Ninth Symphony is not composed of the wood that the violins are made of, nor of the conductor's body, hands and movements, nor of the wood that constitutes the chairs that the players sit on. The symphony is an entity, on one hand, so clear and with such a moving presence, and on the other hand, it does not exist within any of the physical factors that make it exist. The music creates a feeling of time but is not dependent on homogeneous time. Through the music we briefly leave our own personal time to be in a different time in which we believe that the physical and psychic can live together, be one thing and thus the revived feeling of recovery, which is nothing but our own unity with ourselves from a place of clarity and listening, from a place of presence and alertness and renewed sitting within our bodies. The concern of art and science is the abstraction of reality and not the presentation of the instrumental reality as is, the extraction of reality and the presentation of the model but not an exact and ordinary photograph of all the details. Sartre's wonderful example is a painting in which he sees Venice **but there is no actual place in Venice that resembles this painting.** This is the place where the abstract unites with the physical and is the moment of grace in art. I do something with my hands, with my body, with my vocal chords, but this action is not my intention, this action only serves intention which by its definition is not part of the world of objects. Art, like the mind, has at one and the same time, a clear and sharp presence and an elusive quality. Sartre illustrates this in art. "Let us not forget that that which is real is the result of brushstrokes, the adhesiveness of the cloth, the glaze on the paint, but all this is not the object of the aesthetic appreciation, what is 'beautiful' is something that cannot be experienced by sensation (of one of the senses) and is beyond this world." That is to say, it so much exists within us but is not realized as an object in the world. So too the mind, the sensation of the thinking, experiencing self so exists within us but this self is not perceived as a thing (object) in the world. And so, when it is suggested to Sartre to leave the virtual (the world of experience and imagination) for the "real" world he only finds meaningless objects in the actual world. These objects are meaningless because there is no concept of meaning and intention in inanimate nature and consequently the natural sciences are involved with the question of cause and effect and not with the question of meaning and intention, this is empirical science. Ancient "science" dealt with meaning and final cause which was also its weakness - the inability to predict what will happen in point $T1$ when the situation in point $T0$ is known.

We have seen in earlier chapters that mind unites itself when in one period of time, it provides only one meaning to a stimuli received by the nervous system. Perception becomes sensation only when man discovers within himself the possibility of response to the stimuli received by the system. From the likelihood of a response, intention can be aroused - its existence on one hand is so clear (to the one with the intention) and on the other hand, it does not exist as an object in the "world", it is also "out of this world", not to be found in the public domain.

My students discovered new possibilities of insight and experience in the roles they embodied, not because they understood something intellectual or informative and received my interpretations of their role but because I helped them discover within themselves the possibility of uniting the body and the awakening intention. I helped them understand that acting is nothing but the realization of the intention that is clarified in the process of performance. In this process the foreignness of the observer viewing his body from the side does not exist but rather, there is the experience of orientation in which the total self is immersed in a clarifying process and the desire to persevere despite the obstacles. These are the clear signs of the correct actions in both art and science. The clear feeling of the acting I who is in a clarification process, in its actualization, with a clear will and desire to proceed despite the difficulties along the way. Interestingly, Spinoza spoke about identity, between understanding and will. Understanding in the sense of insight of experience, discovering the connection between things, finding the whole via the connection between its parts that is actually one of the ways that science "understands" the world. Thus, both art and science serve man's *a priori* need to discover within himself the possibility of uniting the mind. The teleceptors and the nervous system make it possible for man to see and hear, **but who is it that sees and hears? He is so present and at the same time absent**, this is true for the work of art as well.

Seeing the unity in nature provides man with meaning in making the existence of his mind possible, and thus man becomes part of his environment. The existence of the mind as a clear and distinct entity is decisively significant for survival value, since only with this clarity can man guarantee the continuation of the race; a chaotic and amorphous state cannot guarantee this.

It is interesting that the theory of chaos in physics posits that the world is built as an integration of order and chaos. Something that is predictable with elements that are not predictable beforehand and there are those who claim that the beauty of nature is thus revealed to us. Imagine a rose bush whose leaves and flowers and stems are identical, uniform; how monstrous and ugly and threatening this bush would seem to us. In my opinion, this matter is connected to the predictable and planned elements of the mind, such as: tomorrow at 10:00 o'clock, I will meet this person at this place. Homogeneous time lets us live in the "instrumental world". However, our inner experiential world has its own time, imaginary time that creates things that cannot be predicted beforehand. Accordingly, Sartre said that a great writer is not God, he does not know what will happen with his characters tomorrow, they have their own existence, their own life and the writer is only a mediator to write things down and clarify them. Consequently, there is often sterile intellectualism that

Chapter Seven

doesn't generate anything new in its attempt to understand in advance. This is true in both science and art; education should allow the student his course of **walking towards the unknown** from a clear experience of the one I, with will and desire to continue in the process. This is exactly what the infant does when he teaches himself the basic skills (walking, standing) if adults do not disturb him (see chapter on Experiencing and Learning).

In evolution, development was connected with imagination and not with knowledge or memory. The same primitive creature that in the course of evolution became a complex animal with brain and mind did not do this based on previous knowledge or memory, because he created something that did not exist beforehand. In this sense, science and art at their best are the human continuation of the evolutionary process in that they create something which did not exist beforehand and could not be constructed or envisioned based upon prior knowledge alone. The mind discovers itself while it discovers the world and discovers the world while it discovers itself and as we have already said, according to Sartre, a good play is a play in which, on one hand, the characters reveal themselves and their complexity to us in the happenings of the play, and on the other hand, a gradual revelation of the characters advances what happens in the play.

In every pathological state, this process of discovery and clarification is stopped; in every condition that needs repair, there is a vicious circle in which the "cause is the effect and the effect is the cause" and there is no way of breaking out of this circle, no way of reaching understanding or perhaps more precisely, insight, and therefore there is also no possibility of arriving at clear will, clear desire with the feeling of wakefulness choice and the state of finite mind.

According to Sherrington, the live cell is a harmonious entity in time and space and as we have seen, the mind is also interwoven and cannot be separated from the concepts of time and space. Time is the element that makes the unity of the mind possible. There is no existence to the concept of mind without the concept of time, as we have already seen, because the mind perceives the different data that enters the brain as representing one reality because the observed event occurred in one period of time. The human mind cannot be described in linear terms since one cannot isolate two components and show in a straight line a state of cause and effect in the relations between them; in every experiment the mind will appear as one entity. Someone defined a non-linear form as the measurement of the diagonal of a room; with every step one takes to measure it, the length of the diagonal changes. Imaginary artistic and mental time is created when the person is in a state of search and excitement, needing to experience and understand and discover something that is unpredictable beforehand, exactly what happened in evolution and therefore, being in the state of imaginary time has a sense of free will and wakefulness choice. Being only in homogenous time is one of the symptoms of a pathological state in which time is clutched like a lifesaver is clutched before sinking into the oblivion of the mind. A schizophrenic state, as we have seen, sometimes ends in a vegetative state, in which there is no feeling of time, and the patient sinks into a continuous present. In this state there is apparently a very blurry feeling and experience of the "I that is acting" and there is no feeling of control over the actions from a position of wakefulness.

The meaning and spirit of art is man's continuing search for the possibility of building himself anew every time as an entity in which the physical reality (deterministic, seemingly neutral) and the psychic, abstract unpredictable reality unite, with the possibility of intention and will, two elements that do not exist in the physical reality. In artistic mastery, the person builds himself as a richer whole with the clearer feeling of unity with himself. Here, the principle of unity in multiplicity is fulfilled more fully, not in a bewitched state (like the person who gets angry, for example) but with the feeling of clear presence, the ability to look into oneself and experience what is happening within while at the same time being able to stimulate and inhibit the process. In art, there is a more discerning relationship to the time-space dimension with a more exacting inhibition and the source of satisfaction is the process of refining the intention. Discovery of the grades of mind will also help in clarifying intentions and will eliminate the different parasitic forces that blur the mind and usually serve such needs as praise and recognition that stem from a deep feeling of lack of self-worth.

As we have said, in the process of examining grades of mind, the true intention will become clear as well as the person's attitude to materia. If a person is, for example, in a process of searching for his own worth, the system will not work interactively since this statement contains a contradiction. On one hand, there is aspiration to act, to be in a state of capability and on the other hand, there is a deep feeling of inability and consequently, the search for self-worth from others. In this state, there cannot be a clear feeling of the cohesive active I and a person cannot regulate his own well-being. All the learning process and assimilation of new material in science and art must be done with the teacher seeing the student as being of supreme value and enabling him to face the unknown with a profound feeling of solidarity and interactivity.

Every attempt to force the student into a "desirable" character or to ask for the right answer will only leave him without the vitality of a true happening within himself and without the real ability to act. This attempt actually negates the student's being at any given moment and does not facilitate the basic conditions of solidarity and interactivity. It is important to note here that in assimilating something new, it is not only information that is presented to the student but also the teacher's relationship to the student and the student's relationship to himself. If the student was accustomed to studying in a process that deligitimized him, then whenever he has to digest new material this deligitimization will crop up and not allow the authentic process of assimilation and internalization to occur. In a healthy and true process, there is communication with the teacher and with the environment without harming the integrity of the student, in this state there is a direct and simple looking outside and no preoccupation with the question of how. One of the important questions to ask every student who is in the process of doing his art or research is: **What do you want now or what is the primary thing engaging you now?**

The focus on action need not be expressed in the attempt to focus on the internal listening to one place or thing. Improved action is expressed in the ability to let attention wander freely while acting and functioning, from a dynamic balance that does not exclude any position or possibility. One should remember that skills also include innovativeness and are not an exact mechanical repetition of the identical thing. Therefore, one can say that in true artistic or scientific performance, there is a feeling of volition and inventiveness without the person feeling any inner opposition. **In this state the person creates one reality for himself and a clear feeling of orientation within this reality.** The individual and this reality become one unity, the person no longer looks from the outside and all his different parts are cohesive in one physical and mental space. The artistic experience, similar to sexual orgasm, takes us out of ourselves only to return us to the same primary part within ourselves, but more refreshed and vital and temporarily liberated from the parasitic forces of our "experimental personality".

The natural sciences leave the individual facing a purposeless reality while in art, the individual constructs his own purposeful model.

DR. MOSHE FELDENKRAIS - BIOGRAPHY

Dr. Moshe Feldenkrais was born in 1904 in the Ukrainian town of Slavuta. At the age of 14 he emigrated to Israel (then Palestine) and worked as a construction laborer until the age of 20. In 1925, after graduating from Tel Aviv's first high school, he worked as a cartographer for the British survey office. During this time, he began his studies of self-defense, including Jiu-Jitsu. A soccer injury that he suffered in 1929 would later trigger the development of his method.

Feldenkrais left for France, and during the 1930s lived in Paris where he gained a mechanic and electrical engineering degree from the Ecole des Travaux Publics des Paris, and later his Ph.D. in physics at the Sorbonne. Dr. Moshe Feldenkrais worked at the Radium Institute as a research assistant to Frédéric Joliot-Curie, the nuclear physicist and chemist who later won the Nobel Prize.

In 1933, after meeting with Jigoro Kano, the founder of judo, he began studying it seriously, and in 1936 he became the first European to earn a black belt in judo from the Kodokan Academy in Tokyo. He gained his 2nd black belt degree in 1938, and founded the first Jiu-Jitsu Club of Paris and one of the first in Europe, training the J.J.C.F. in France during its first 10 years of activity. This club, which has branches all over France, now has over one million members.

When World War II broke, Dr. Feldenkrais was drafted to the National Center for Scientific Research (C.N.R.S.), and just before Paris was conquered in 1940, he fled to England. He served as a science officer in the British Admiralty until 1946, working on anti-submarine warfare, and his work on improving sonar led to 6 patents in France and England for his invention.

When teaching self-defense techniques to his fellow servicemen, he re-aggravated his knee injury, which urged him to intently explore and develop self-rehabilitation techniques that later became part of his method.

After leaving the Admiralty, Feldenkrais lived and worked in the private industry in London, and thanks to his self-rehabilitation he was able to continue his Judo practice. As a member of the International Judo Committee, he began studying Judo systematically, incorporating the knowledge he gained through his self-rehabilitation. In 1949 he published the first book on the Feldenkrais method, Body and Mature Behavior. During this period, he studied the work of G.I. Gurdjieff (founder of The Fourth Way), F. Matthias Alexander (Founder of Alexander Technique), and William Bates (known for the Bates Method of eye exercises). He also traveled to Switzerland to study with German musician and educator, Heinrich Jacoby.

In 1951, Dr. Feldenkrais returned to the recently-formed state of Israel, and having directed the Israeli Army Department of Electronics for a few years, he finally settled in Tel Aviv where he began teaching his method full-time. In 1957, he gave lessons in the Feldenkrais method to David Ben-Gurion, Israel's Prime Minister, and became widely known after Ben-Gurion, who was then over 70, posed for the press while standing on his head.

Dr. Feldenkrais founded The Feldenkrais Institute for the Research of Movement and its Perfection. Among his students were presidents, prime ministers and ambassadors, scientists, conductors and actors, and men and women from all around the world.

Throughout the 1960s, 1970s, and into the 1980s, Dr. Feldenkrais presented his method in Europe and North America, and also began to train teachers, so that they could, in their own turn, present his work to others. He trained the first group of 12 teachers in the method from 1969-1971 in Tel Aviv, and over the course of four summers in the years 1975-1978, he trained 65 teachers in San Francisco. In 1980, 235 students began his teacher-training course at Hampshire College in Amherst, Massachussets, but unfortunately, he was not able to complete the course due to illness in 1981.

Dr. Feldenkrais published twenty titles in 12 languages, including Japanese and Portuguese, about autosuggestion, Judo, and his method of training the consciousness and coordinating body and mind.

Among his most important books are:
1) *The Elusive Obvious* – Basic Feldenkrais
2) *The Potent Self* – A Guide to Spontaneity
3) *Improving Ability* – Theory and Practice